MORE THAN A
Cookbook

INCLUDES RECIPES, WORKOUTS + MORE!

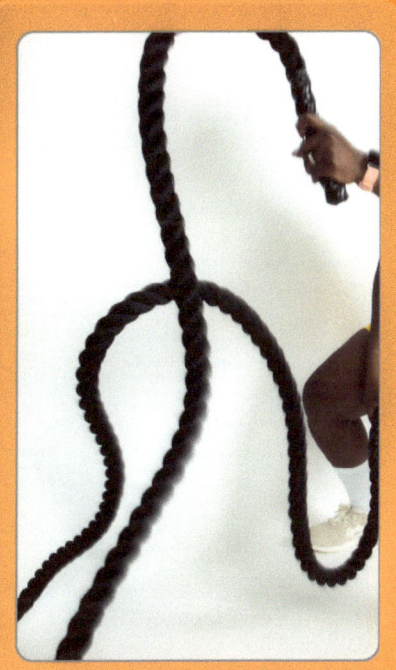
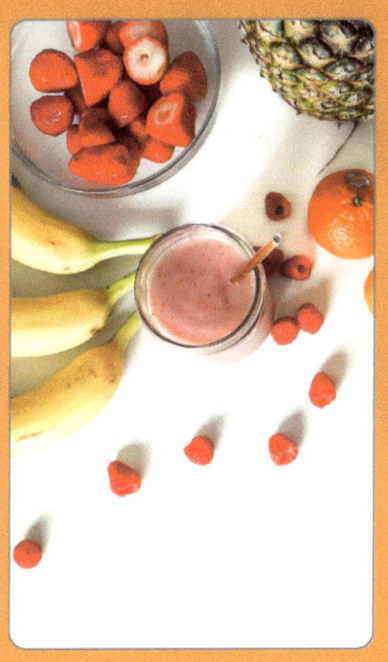
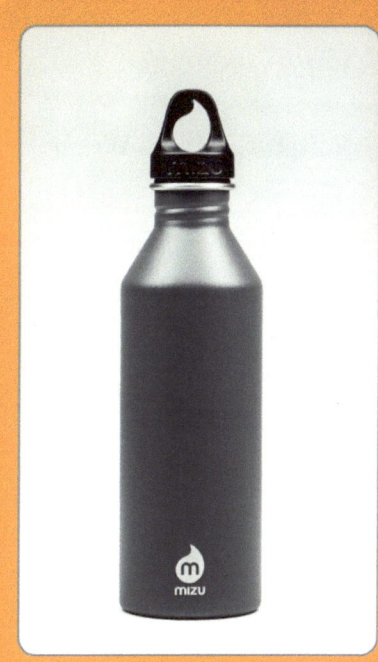

MORE THAN A *Cookbook*

Copyright © 2023 Desarae Stills

All rights reserved.

Although the author have made every effort to ensure that the information in this book was correct at press time, the author does not assume and hereby disclaim any liability to any party for any loss, damage, or disruption caused by errors or omissions, whether such errors or omissions result from negligence, accident, or any other cause.

This book is not intended as a substitute for medical advice of physicians. The reader should regularly consult a physician in matters relating to his/her health and particularly with respect to any symptoms that may require diagnosis or medical attention.

No parts of this book may be reproduced in any form or by any electronic or mechanical means, including information storage in retrieval systems, without written permission from the author, except in the case of a reviewer, who may quote brief passages embodied in critical articles or in a review.

ISBN: 979-8-9883457-4-9

Editor: Crystal S. Wright

10 9 8 7 6 5 4 3 2 1

Printed in the United States

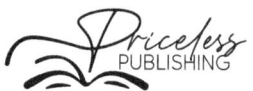

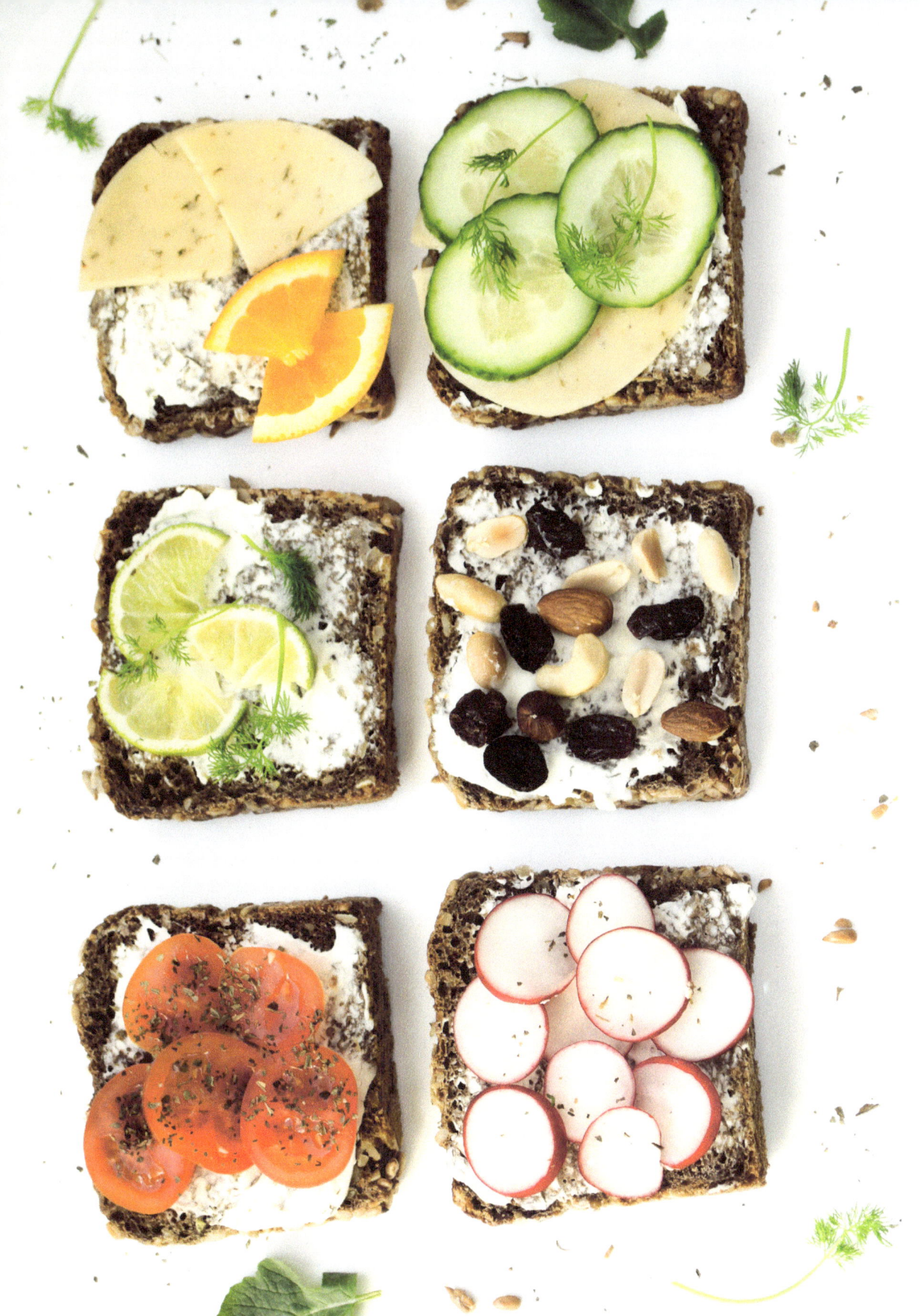

Contents

INTRODUCTION | **1**

FRUITY ALMOND BUTTER TOAST | **3**

HEALTH TIME MANAGEMENT + ORGANIZATION TIPS | **5**

AVOCADO TOAST | **9**

21 MINUTES RULE | **11**

AUNTIE'S CHICKPEA ORZO SALAD | **13**

SMART GOALS FOR IMPROVING HEALTH | **17**

BANANA TUNA FISH | **23**

MINDSET | **26**

BLUEBERRY SWEET | **29**

BEAUTY + EXERCISE | **31**

MEAL PREPPING | **33**

CREATE A RECIPE | **34**

CORE EXCERCISES | **39**

GLUTE BRIDGES | **40**

FRONT PLANK | 41

SIDE PLANK | 42

BUFFALO CHICKEN QUESADIILLA | 43

LEAN BEEFY STUFFED POTATO | 47

BIOLOGICAL CRAVINGS | 50

CRANBERRY OATMEAL COOKIES | 51

TREADMILL WORKOUT | 54

SMOTHERED BONELESS CHICKEN & VEGGIES | 55

BOOTCAMP | 59

PUMPKIN SEED & ALMONDS ROASTED | 63

CHOICES | 65

SWEET AVOCADO SALSA | 67

TIPS I USE FOR VACATION | 70

CUCUMBER & CITRUS INFUSED WATER | 71

SLEEP | 73

FROM THE AUTHOR | 77

Introduction

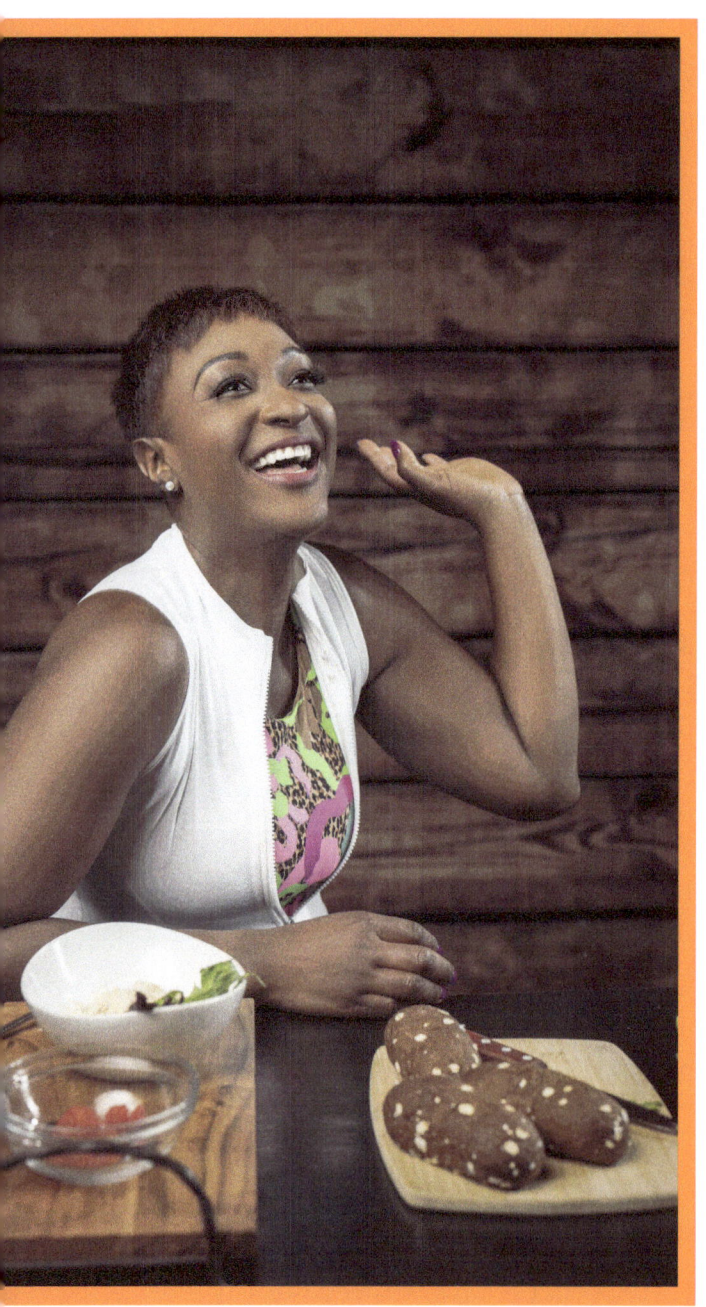

DEAR READER,

As you use this book for more than its recipes, I pray that it moves you closer to improved total health.

I hope this book allows you to feel more confident in yourself, as well as hopeful and realistic about your health journey. I hope you learn how to take charge of your total health and find recipes that you'll enjoy. Finally, I hope you pay it forward by sharing something that you learned with someone else.

May you find joy in movement, and fueling your body with healthy, essential items. I hope you are encouraged and inspired to be the best version of yourself. It's not an accident that you have this book. Trust the process. Dream big. Be consistent. You have more than you know at your fingertips. The ingredients you need to live a healthy life are already inside of you. Now it's up to you to serve it.

BE BLESSED,

Desi

FRUITY ALMOND BUTTER *Toast*

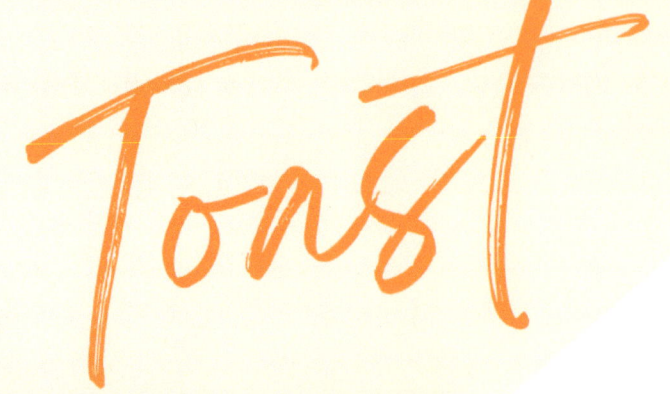

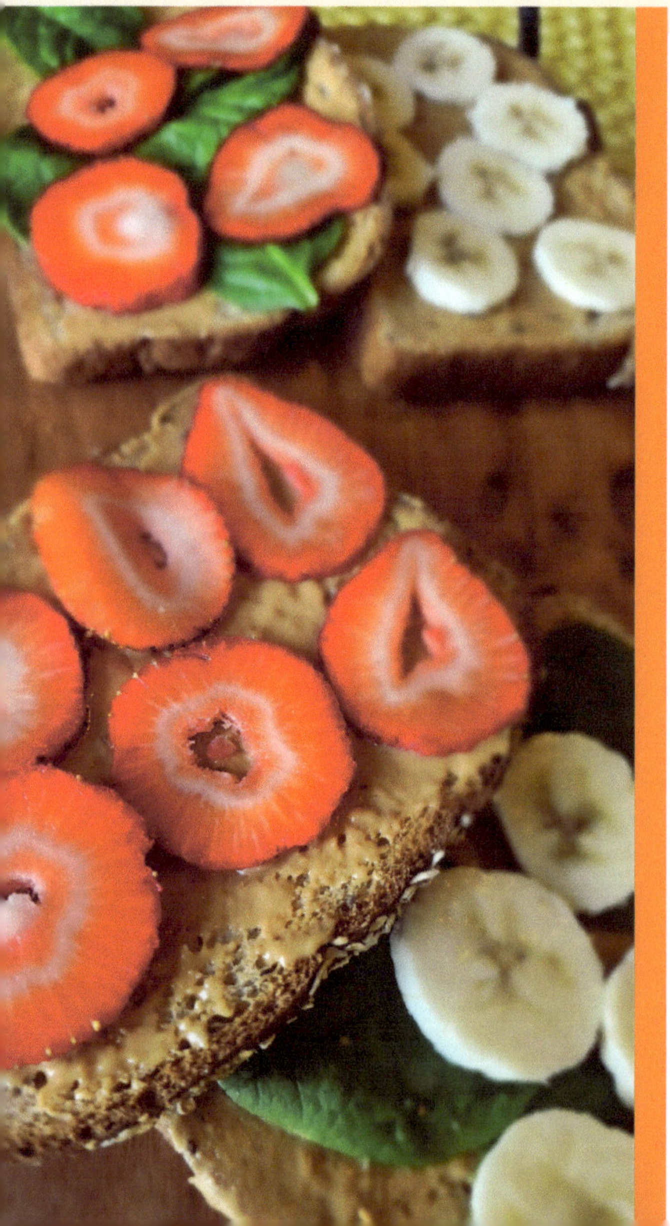

READY IN: 5 MINUTES

SERVING SIZE: 1

INGREDIENTS

- ✓ 1 Slice of wheat bread
- ✓ ¼ cup of Strawberries or ¼ of a banana
- ✓ ¼ cup of Spinach
- ✓ About 1 tbsp of unsweetened almond butter

PREPARATION

1. Wash all produce.
2. Pat fruit with a paper towel. Put fruit on a cutting board and thinly slice. Place fruit in a bowl and set it to the side.
3. Pat dry spinach with a paper towel, place in a bowl and set it to the side.
4. *Optional:* Toast bread.
5. Put bread on a separate plate and spread almond butter on it.
6. Place the spinach on the bread.
7. Finally, add thinly sliced fruit.

TIPS

This is my favorite quick breakfast option. It's great when time is limited. It can be prepared at home, at the office, at school, or even in the car. This recipe can also serve as a great snack for pre-workout or post-workout.

HEALTH TIME MANAGEMENT + ORGANIZATION *Tips*

✓ At the end of each week, I look at my schedule for the upcoming week and plan. I decide which days I will go to the gym and which days I will do meal prep. These are factored into my roles working a 9-5, being a wife and mother, and having a social life. Naturally, I also plan on which days I will eat out and decide on possible restaurant options. I go as far as looking at the menu ahead of time to know my options.

It's important to note that despite our best plans, things happen. My thought process is that if I stick to my plan 80% of the time, when I don't, there will be little to no negative effect on my body or health goals.

Also, plan according to your lifestyle. My lifestyle includes gatherings with my loved ones, with food and drinks sometimes. Currently, I allow myself a *shift* meal, that is, a meal that does not have any restrictions twice a week but it cannot be two consecutive days. I also allow myself 1-2 days of rest from physical activity each week.

When I eat a shift meal (eat what I want), the following day I will exercise plus my meals are typically healthy and I will eat within a calorie deficit 1-2 days following the day I have a shift meal . That is, low carb, no added sugar, whole grain, with lean meat.

✓ I pick out my office clothes for two or more days at the start of the week.

✓ I also do meal-prep. I do it at the start of the week for 2-3 days, and again mid-week (or when time permits) for the remainder of the week.

✓ I also have a calendar on my phone and desktop that I use to plan by the weeks and months. I prioritize my 80/20 eating rule for birthdays, celebrations, and vacations. 80% of the time I eat lean protein, fruits, vegetables, whole grains, and limited added sugar. The other 20% of the time I eat what I want (shift meal).

✓ If I know I'm going out and I will not be eating healthier option foods, every other meal for that day, both what I eat before and after, must be foods that have positive effects on my body.

Example: I am going to Cancun in June. I started making changes to my normal way of eating and exercise as of December. For the last couple of months, I've maintained my normal eating and exercise schedule (80% foods low in carbs, no added sugar, fruits, vegetables and whole grains and 20% is my one shift meal twice a week). The reason for this is because the S.M.A.R.T body goals that I have for Cancun require me to make some dietary changes. It is important to identify what it takes to accomplish your desired goals by a certain time frame. We will discuss S.M.A.R.T. goals later in this book.

PLAN, PLAN, PLAN!

Even if you can't get *everything* done, you can get *something* done and that's more than doing *nothing*. I make planning for meal prep and working out a priority in my life, just as brushing my teeth and putting gas in my car. My health is a full-time job. It's my responsibility to take care of my body.

Trust the Process

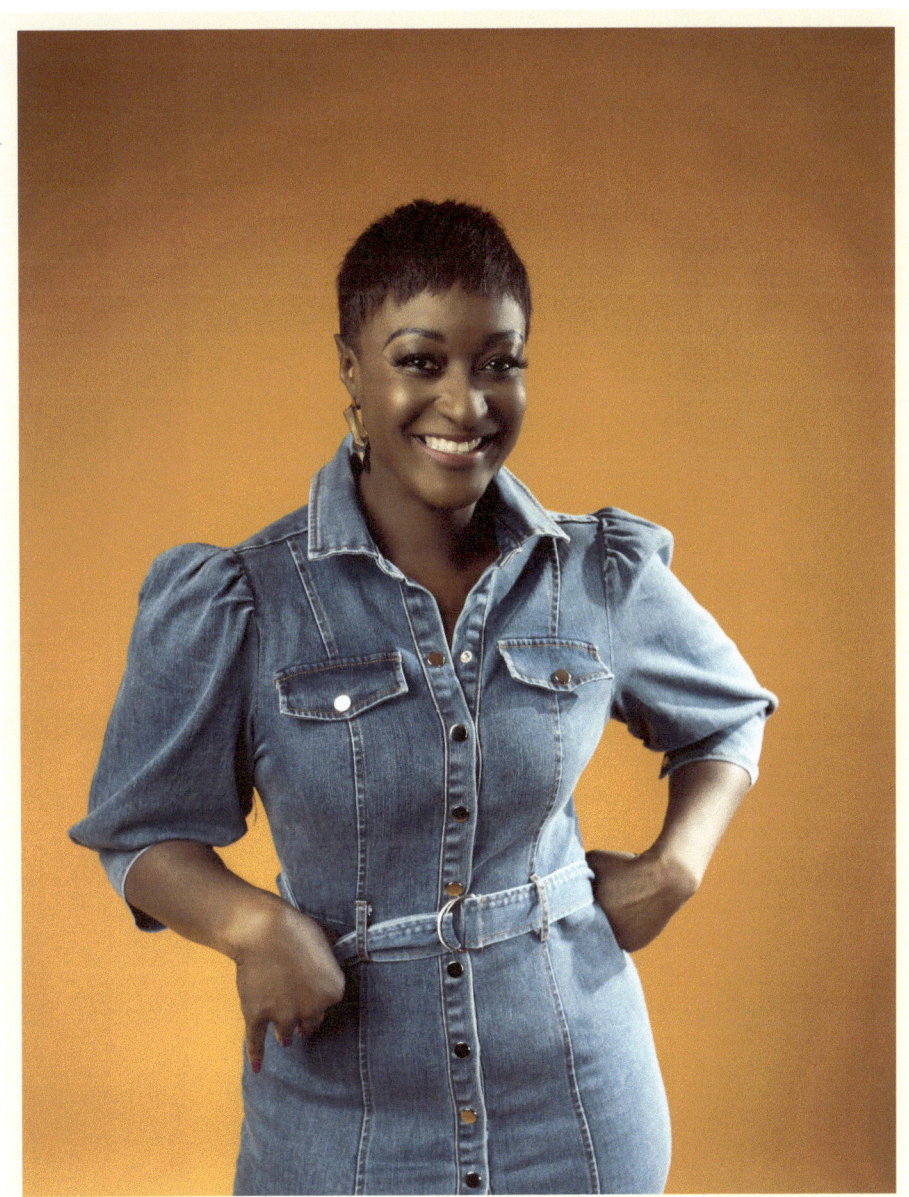

AVOCADO *Toast*

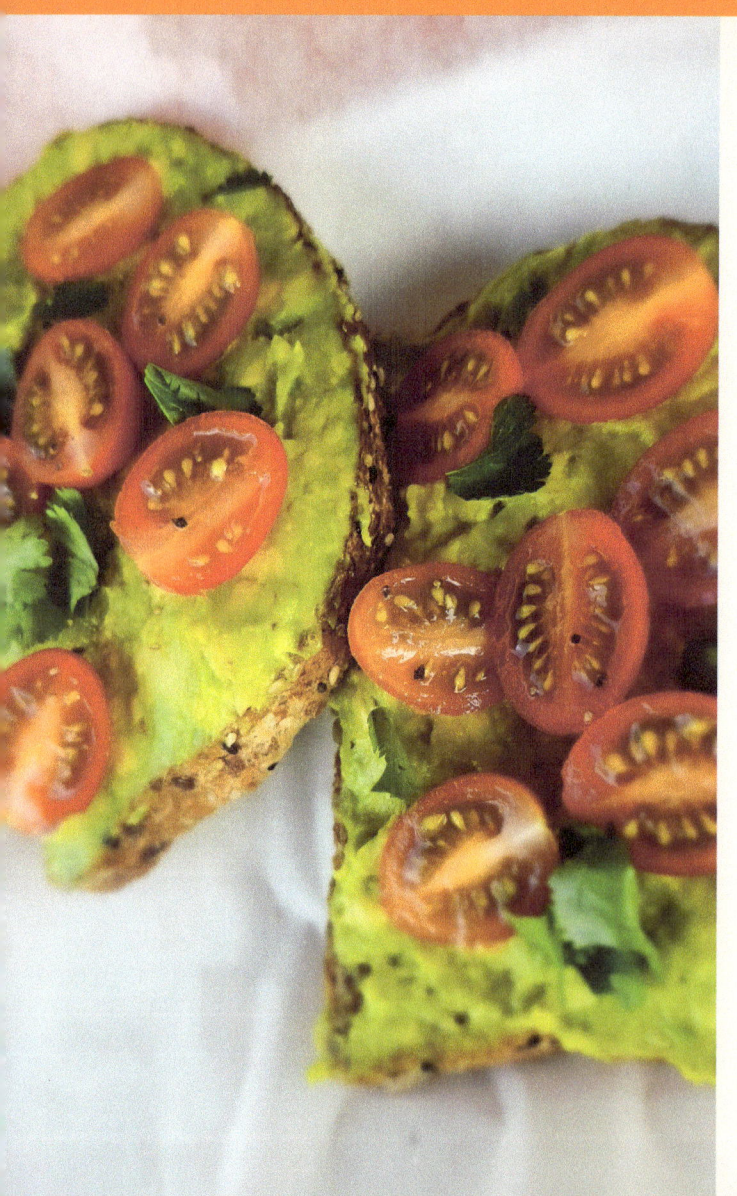

READY IN: **5 MINUTES**

SERVING SIZE: **2**

INGREDIENTS

- ✓ 1 Avocado
- ✓ 5 Grape size tomatoes
- ✓ Pinch of salt
- ✓ 1 tsp Lime juice
- ✓ ¼ cup Parsley, chopped
- ✓ Pinch of pepper
- ✓ 2 Slices of whole grain wheat bread

PREPARATION

1. Toast bread and put it to the side.
2. Rinse all produce.
3. Split the avocado in half and spoon the middle into a bowl. Mash with a fork and put to the side.
4. Slice tomatoes and add to the bowl of smashed avocado.
5. Add parsley, salt, pepper, and lime juice to the bowl and mix.
6. Spread the avocado mix onto the bread and serve.

TIPS

This is a great breakfast, lunch, or snack option. As a breakfast option, you can add 1 scrambled egg on top of the avocado mix. As a lunch option you can add avocado mix to a salad and have wheat bread on the side.

21 MINUTES *Rule*

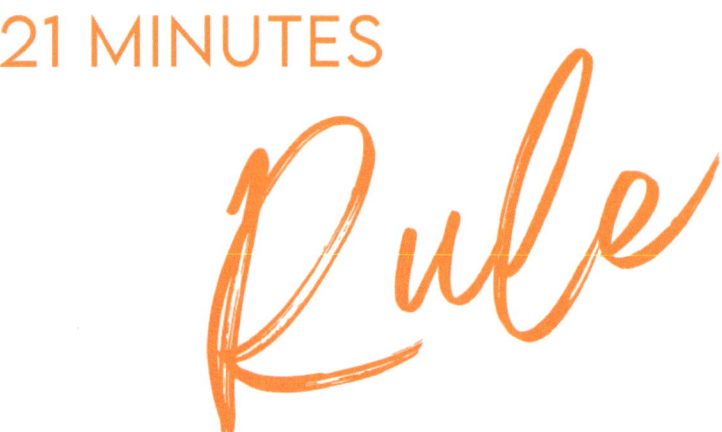

When I eat, I try to only eat one serving per meal.

I wait 21 minutes after the first serving, and if I'm still hungry, I will have a second serving of food. I drink at least 8oz of water.

Often, I find that I'm not hungry after the first serving but that I just wanted a second serving.

The desire to want more than we need can be related to so many aspects of our life. If we just stop, and think before we react and trust that God has given us more than enough to live purposely it can make all the difference in our tomorrow.

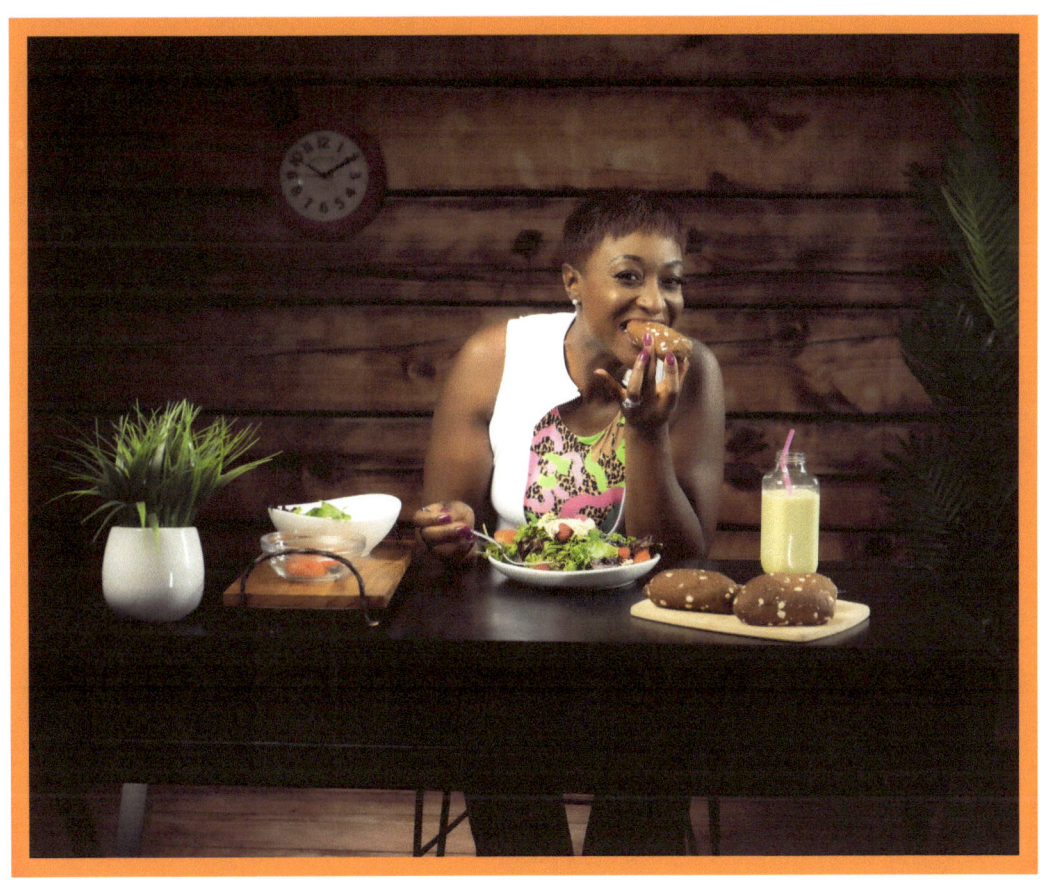

AUNTIE'S CHICKPEA ORZO *Salad*

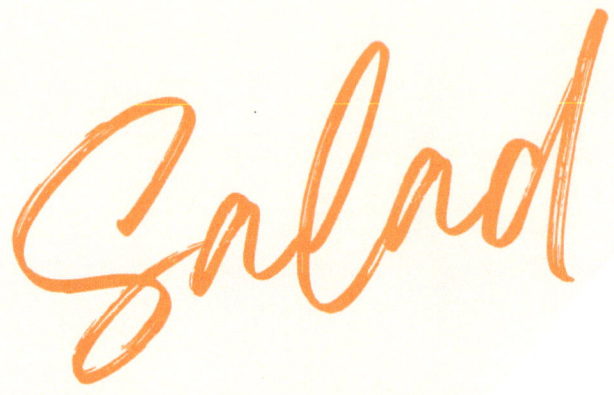

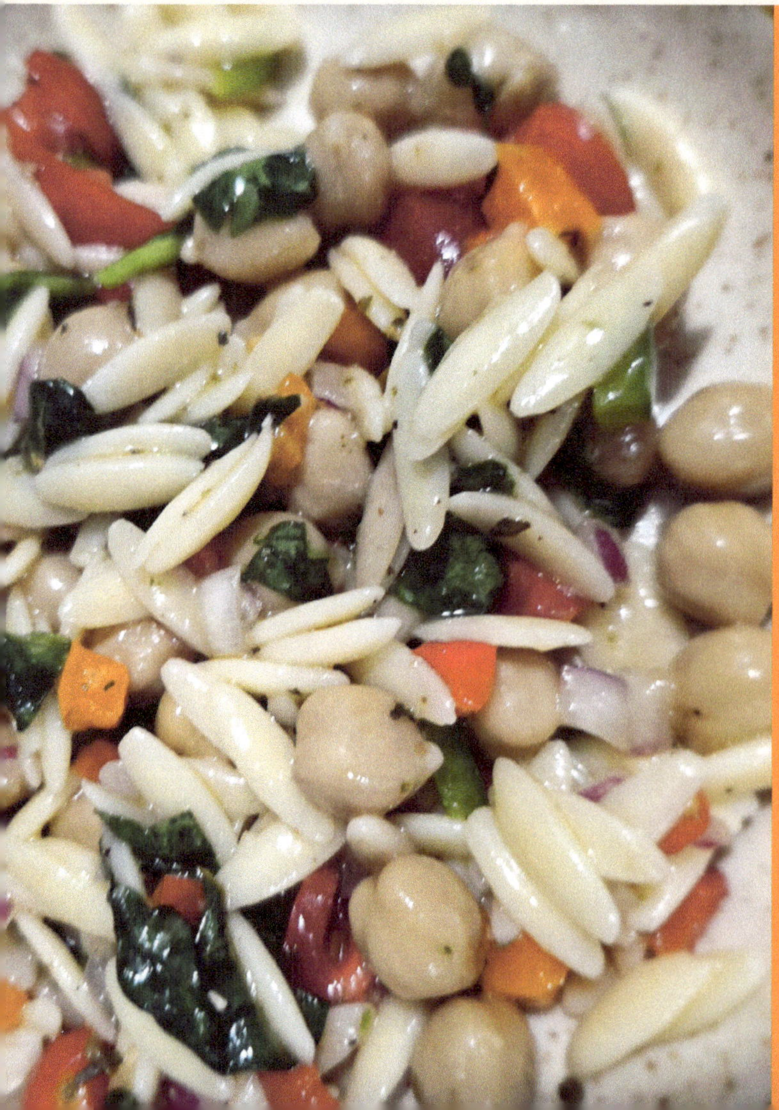

READY IN: 30 MINUTES

SERVING SIZE: 4

INGREDIENTS FOR ORZO SALAD

- ✓ 1 ½ cups of Orzo
- ✓ ½ Green pepper chopped
- ✓ ½ cup Red bell pepper chopped
- ✓ ⅓ cup Red onion diced
- ✓ ½ cup of Spinach
- ✓ 1 cup Cooked chickpea drained and rinsed
- ✓ ⅓ cup Chopped fresh basil
- ✓ ¼ teaspoon of Sea salt and black pepper
- ✓ 2 cups of halved Cherry tomatoes
- ✓ Olive oil/Avocado oil

INGREDIENTS FOR GREEK DRESSING

- ✓ ¼ cup of Extra virgin oil/Avocado oil
- ✓ 1 teaspoon Honey or agave
- ✓ 2-4 tablespoons Freshly squeezed lemon
- ✓ 3 tablespoons of Red wine vinegar
- ✓ ¼ Sea salt
- ✓ ½ teaspoon Dried oregano
- ✓ ¼ Dijon mustard
- ✓ Fresh ground pepper
- ✓ 1 Garlic clove

PREPARATION FOR ORZO SALAD

1. Cook Orzo according to package directions. Drain Orzo and toss in a little Olive oil/Avocado Oil.

2. Dice and chop vegetables.

3. In a large bowl toss, Orzo, spinach, red onions, basil tomatoes, green and red peppers.

PREPARATION FOR GREEK DRESSING

1. In a small bowl whisk together oregano, olive oil/avocado oil, garlic, vinegar, mustard, agave/honey, fresh lemon, sea salt, and pepper.

TIPS

The dressing can be used alone on a salad or a marinade for meat. Pasta can be enjoyed chilled or warm.

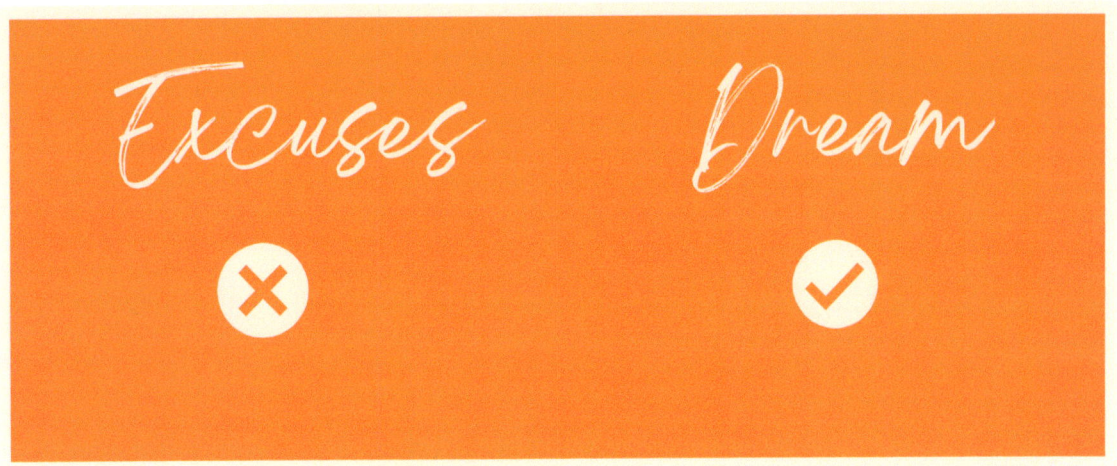

...In order for your dreams to come true,
your dreams must be better than your excuses.
If your excuses are bigger than your dreams,
your dreams will not come true.

SMART GOALS FOR IMPROVING *Health*

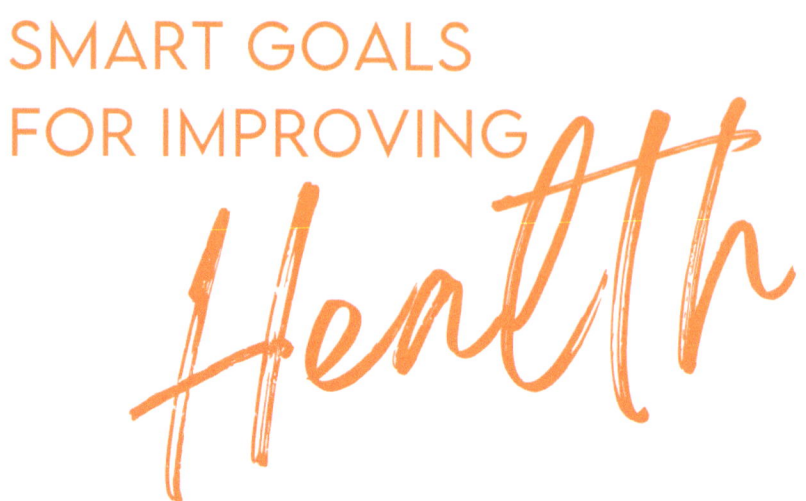

This section is a template to help you create S.M.A.R.T. goals for your health journey.

S.M.A.R.T. goals are **S**pecific, **M**easurable, **A**chievable, **R**elevant and **T**ime-bound. It is more likely that you will achieve your goal when it is a SMART one. Review the information below and fill in information about your goals as you go along.

Be **SPECIFIC**. Think of something specific you want to accomplish that would improve your health (physical or mental). For example, a goal to "feel better about myself" could be too broad and require specific breakdowns of what feeling good means to you.

Answering questions such as *what, where, who,* and *which* will help you to be specific about your goals.

Example: I have an upcoming trip to Cancun in 6 months. My specific goals are that I want to reduce my waistline by 4 inches and the appearance of cellulite on my thighs by then.

WRITE DOWN YOUR SPECIFIC GOAL(S).

_____
_____
_____
_____
_____
_____
_____
_____
_____
_____
_____

MEASURE the success of accomplishing this goal, or moving closer to it. Your goal must be one that can be measured or assessed in some way. If it isn't, how will you know you have achieved it? How will you know how close or far you are from your target?

Goals such as "feeling better" or "looking sexier" are examples of goals that are not specific enough and cannot be measured.

Do some research. Consult with a licensed professional such as a medical doctor, therapist, personal trainer, or nutrition coach on how to accomplish your goal, and determine how to identify progress. (For example: lab work, physical assessment, mental clarity, body weight, etc).

Example: I measured my waistline at the beginning of the six-month period, and noted the measurement. I can measure again every month and note the measurement. This way, I can look at the figures and measure my progress over time.

For the cellulite, I took pictures of my thighs. I can photograph the same sections every month and note the measurement. This way, I can look at the photos and measure my progress over time.

WRITE DOWN HOW YOU WILL MEASURE YOUR PROGRESS AS YOU PURSUE YOUR SPECIFIC GOAL(S).

_____
_____
_____
_____
_____
_____
_____
_____
_____
_____
_____
_____

This is where you answer *how* you plan to **ACHIEVE** this specific, measurable goal. Do you have time to exercise twice a week? Do you have the funds to hire a personal trainer? Can you realistically fast from social media?

WRITE DOWN HOW YOU PLAN TO ACHIEVE THIS SPECIFIC MEASURABLE GOAL.

Example: I hired both a personal trainer and a nutritionist. They created a six-month plan for my diet and exercise so that on a daily, weekly, and month basis I would know what to do to move closer to my goal.

_____

_____

_____

_____

_____

_____

_____

_____

_____

_____

_____

Your goal should be **RELEVANT** to you. Be real with yourself. The goal(s) should align with your identity and other goals. Is this goal important to you, or is it important to your spouse or parents or friends? How will you feel once you accomplish this goal? Are you pursuing this goal for yourself or to keep up with a trend, impress people on social media or make someone jealous?

If your goal is not relevant to you, it is unlikely to be motivated to achieve it. Even if you achieve it, you will not be able to maintain the results.

Example: I have a genuine desire to improve and maintain total health. Reducing the size of my waist and the appearance of cellulite ties into that larger goal. Even after my trip to Cancun, it's likely that I will maintain the results because it is important to me and aligned with my larger goals.

WRITE DOWN WHY THE GOAL(S) IS/ARE IMPORTANT TO YOU.

_____
_____
_____
_____
_____
_____
_____
_____
_____
_____
_____
_____

Set a **TIMEFRAME** that is realistic. Rome wasn't built overnight. Notice that my example includes a timeframe. Without a timeframe, you are chasing a moving target. A timeframe gives you a sense of urgency and will help you to feel motivated as you move closer to your deadline. Regardless of the timeframe for achieving your goal, break it up into smaller chunks, based on when you will measure.

Example: My timeframe is six months. I am aiming to see a reduction in my waistline of at least an inch each month when I measure. I am aiming to see less visibility of the cellulite on my thighs each month when I take a new picture.

WRITE DOWN THE TIMEFRAME IN WHICH YOU WANT TO ACHIEVE YOUR GOAL(S), AND TIMEFRAMES IN WHICH YOU WILL CHECK FOR PROGRESS.

_____
_____
_____
_____
_____
_____
_____
_____
_____
_____
_____
_____

Keep in mind that most health and mindset goals take time to accomplish. However, the purpose of this exercise is to set goals, create a plan and believe that you can do it. Every day that you put in work toward your goals you are closer than you were the day before.

TRUST THE PROGRESS AND KEEP GOING.

BANANA TUNA
Fish

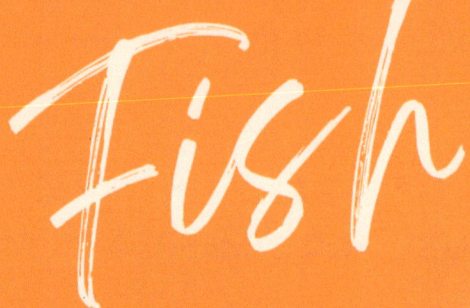

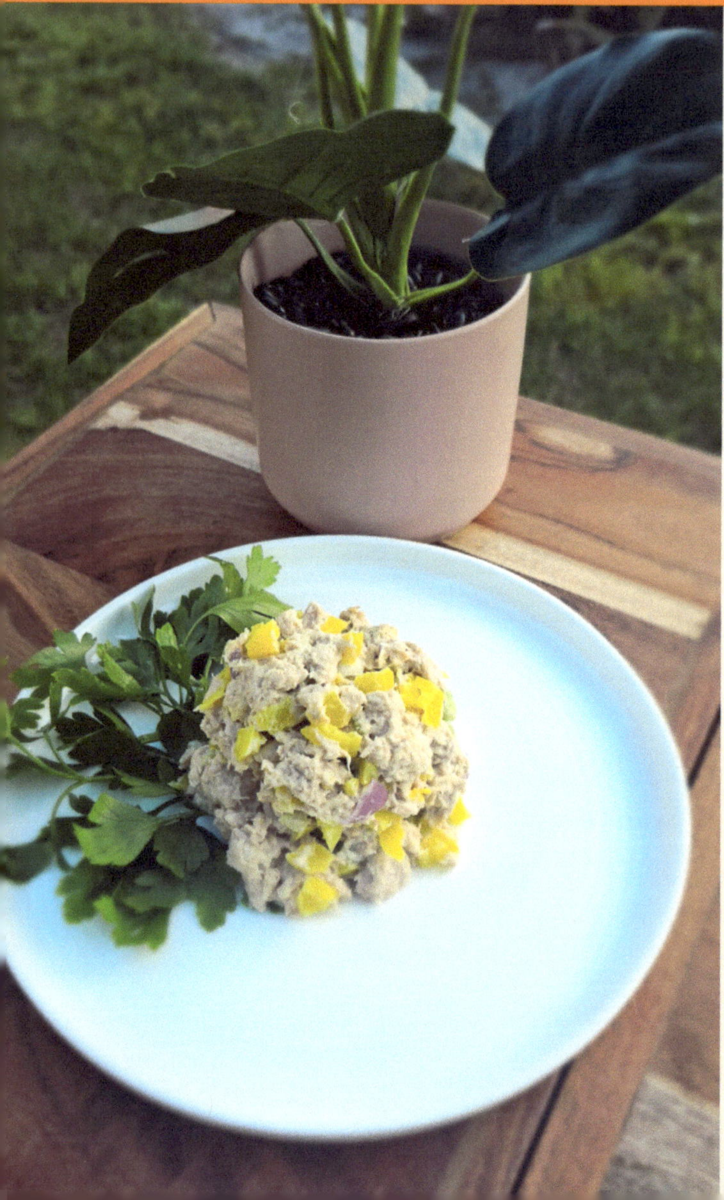

READY IN: 15 MINUTES

SERVING SIZE: 2-3

INGREDIENTS

- ✓ Boiled eggs *(optional)*
- ✓ ¼ cup to ⅓ cup Avocado mayo
- ✓ 1 tbsp Mustard or Dijon mustard
- ✓ 1/8 tsp Sea salt
- ✓ ⅛ tsp Pepper
- ✓ ¼ cup Banana peppers, chopped
- ✓ 8 oz of chunk light tuna in water, drained (canned)
- ✓ ¼ cup of Red onions
- ✓ ¼ cup Green onions
- ✓ 1 Diced celery

PREPARATION

1. Finely mince green onions, red onions, and chop banana peppers then mix all into a bowl and put to the side. *Optional:* Boil 2 eggs, chop the eggs, small to medium size, and place into the bowl of onions and banana peppers.
2. Drain tuna and add to the bowl of onions, and banana peppers to make tuna mixture.
3. Combine avocado mayo, mustard, salt, and pepper into the bowl of tuna mixture.
4. Put Tuna fish in a storage container and place in the refrigerator for at least 30 minutes to chill. Serve cold.

TIPS

The banana pepper adds a nice crunch and little kick. This dish goes great on top of a spring mix salad or as a Tuna sandwich paired with homemade potato chips.

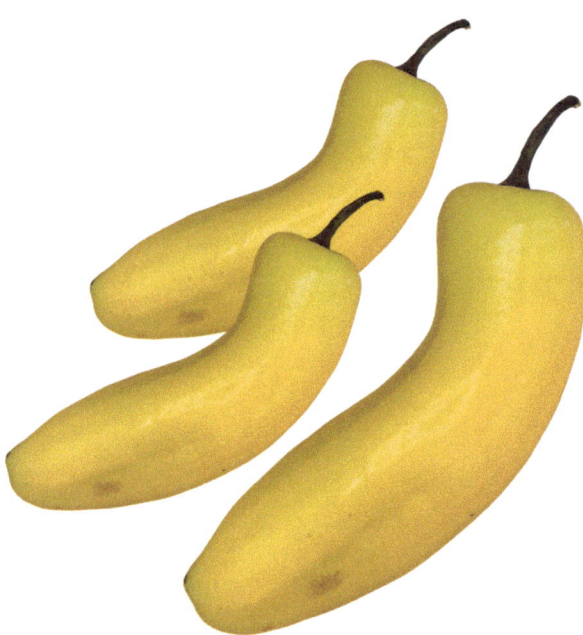

Mindset

Our beliefs affect whether we succeed in something we want. If this holds true, then changing our beliefs, which relates to our mindset, can have a major effect on our lives. Some people are naturally confident while others struggle to believe in themselves.

Although I don't currently struggle with low self-esteem, there have been plenty of times in my life when I had to give myself a pep-talk. I've had to encourage myself. How did I do that? I would confront my fears and flaws head on and take steps to overcome them. I apply what I learn. Finally, I reassure myself I can do all things through God who strengthens me, and I believe it!

Understand that not having the answer today, doesn't mean you won't have the answer *tomorrow*.

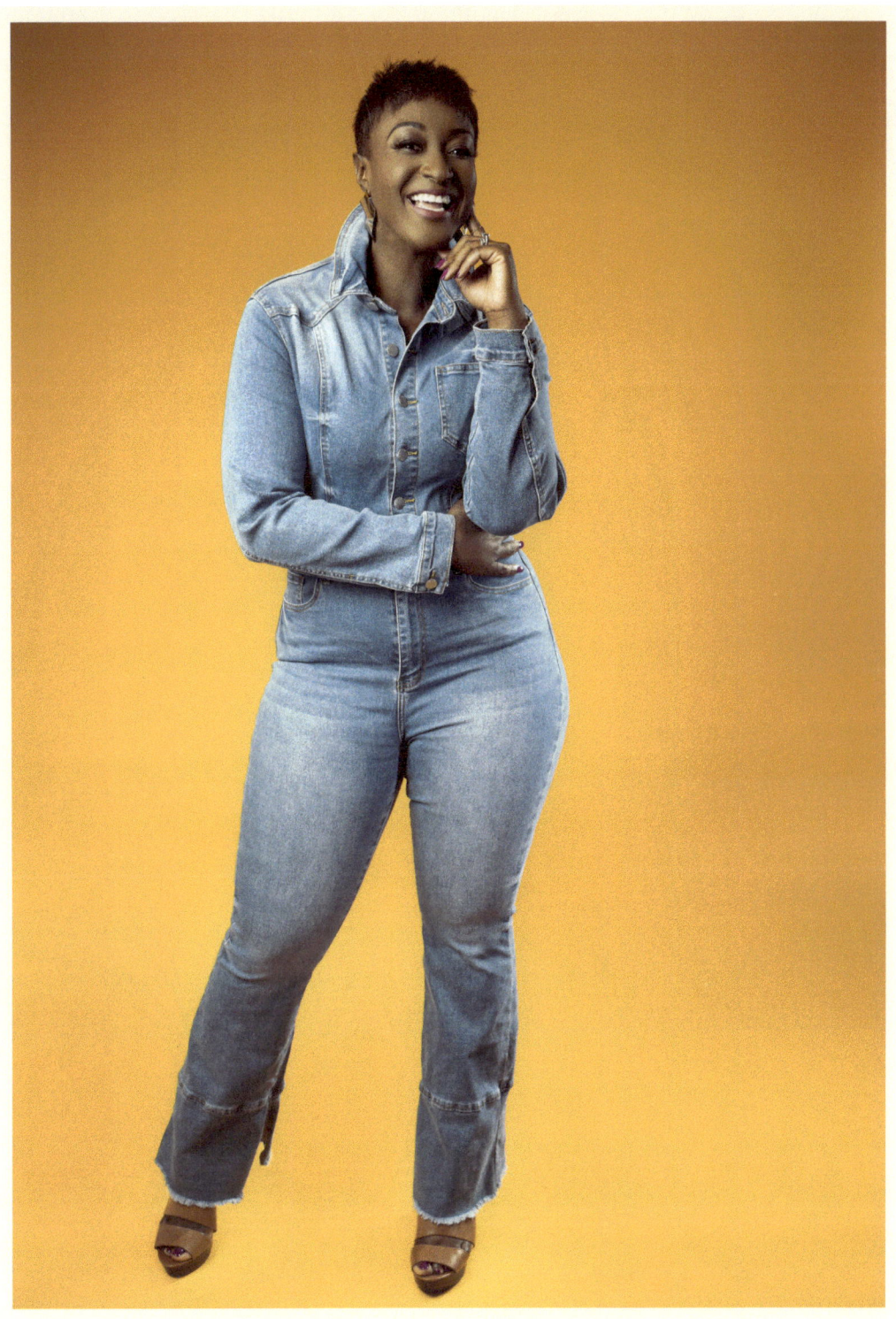

BLUEBERRY *Sweet*

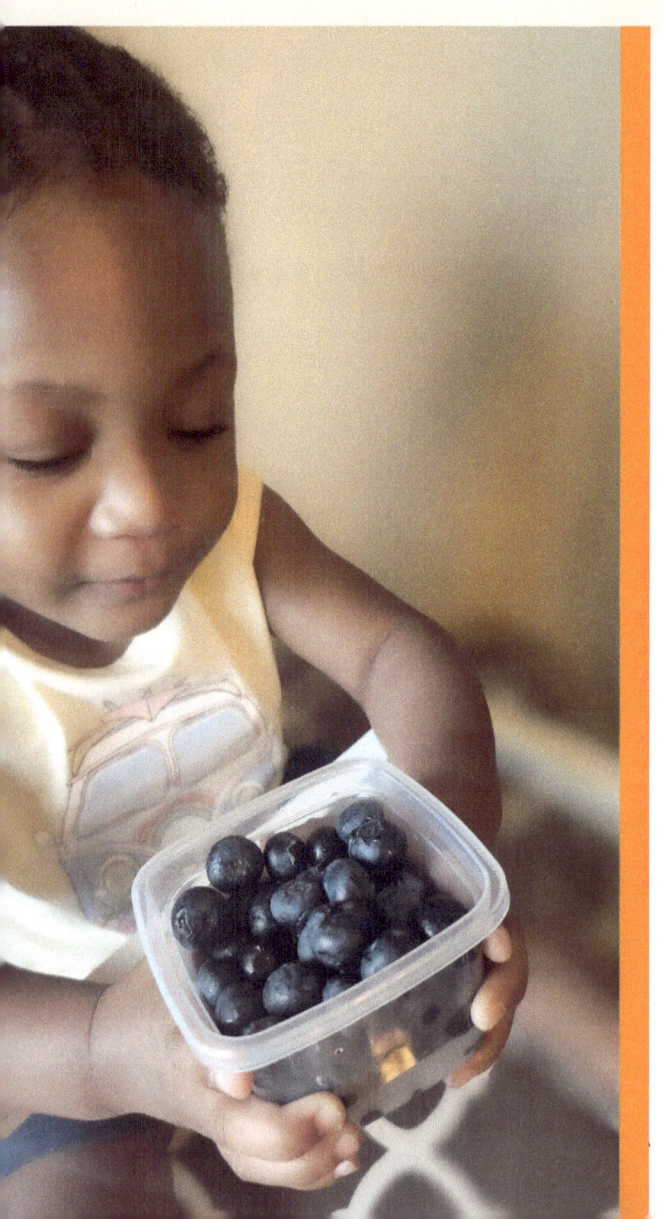

AN EASY TREAT...

A sweet tooth treat that I keep in my freezer is frozen blueberries.

I will take ½ cup to 1 cup of blueberries, rinse them, then pat dry with a paper towel. Put blueberries in a freezer-safe container and let it freeze for about 4 hours to overnight.

This snack is ready to eat directly out of the freezer. The ice coldness of the blueberry brings out the natural sweetness and allows the taste to linger in the mouth. It is perfect for those days and nights when you crave sweets.

My young nieces also love this cool treat.

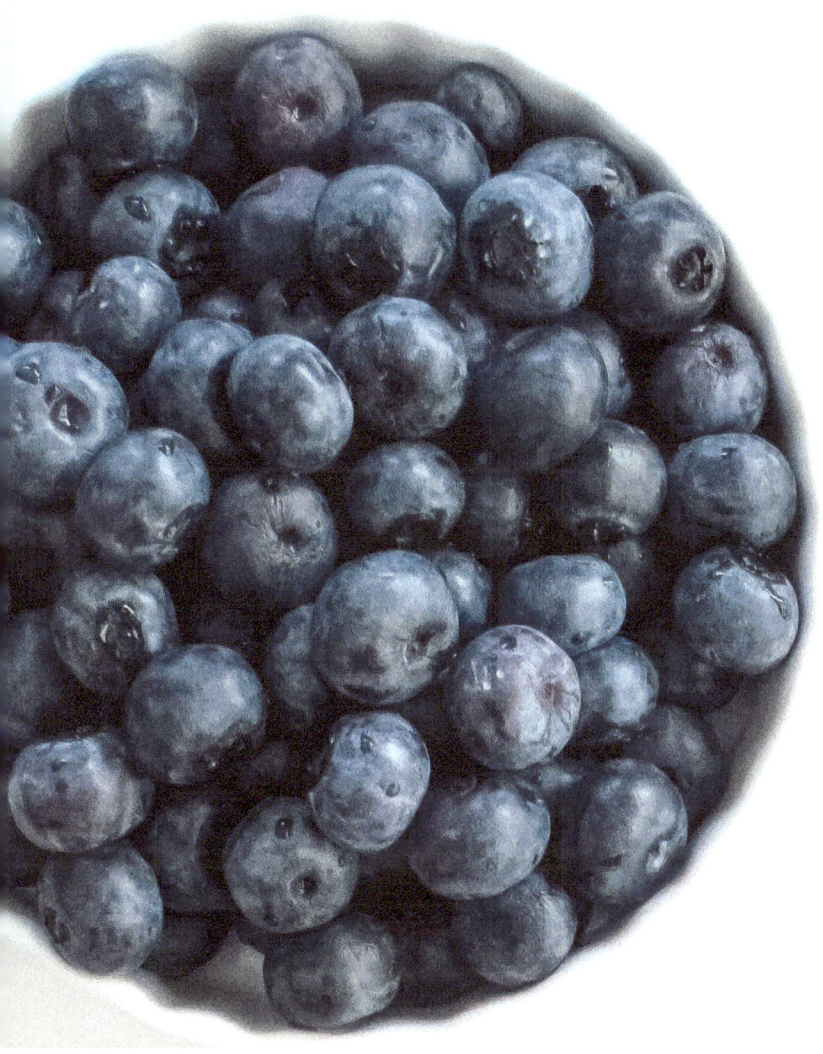

Beauty + Exercise

Like so many of us, I used to shy away from exercise because of the sweating process. For me, I did not want my hair to be sweaty and my skin would burn from sweat. I learned that what I put in my body plays a huge factor in how my skin reacts to the toxins coming out through sweat. As I began to limit my intake of added sugar, eat more vegetables, and drink more water, my skin visibly improved. I no longer experienced irritation from sweating, and I learned how to protect my hair.

I am not a medical or cosmetology professional. It is always a positive to consult with a professional if you are experiencing any kind of discomfort during exercise, whether it is body aches or irritation of the skin.

Below are a few things I do to protect my hair and skin when exercising:

DRINK WATER.
Water hydrates the body, which benefits your skin. My skin has a natural glow with no irritation when exercising when I'm hydrated. I drink at least 20 ounces of water 30 minutes before exercising, 10 ounces while exercising and 20 ounces right after exercising.

CONSULTED AN ESTHETICIAN AND DERMATOLOGIST.
I learned about my skin type and how to care for my skin before and after exercising. This included recommendations for skin care products and natural remedies. Like using a headband or satin scarf hair wrap when exercising. A satin hair wrap helps minimize sweat

build-up on my scalp and absorb some of the sweat from dripping from my head to my face and eyes.

BLOW DRYING MY HAIR.
I do this immediately after exercising, with the dryer on a cool setting. This practice has reduced sweat gathering in my hair roots long after working out.

SHOWER SHORTLY AFTER EXERCISING.
When I shower within 1 hour of exercising, I notice the boost in my muscle recovery and my skin all over is not irritated.

WOOD THERAPY.
With wood therapy I have experienced benefits of toxic release and less water retention. I do this once every 6-8 weeks.

There is no ONE solution for all lifestyles, skin, and body types. Listen to your body, consult with professionals, and do your research. Find a process that works for you.

Meal Prepping

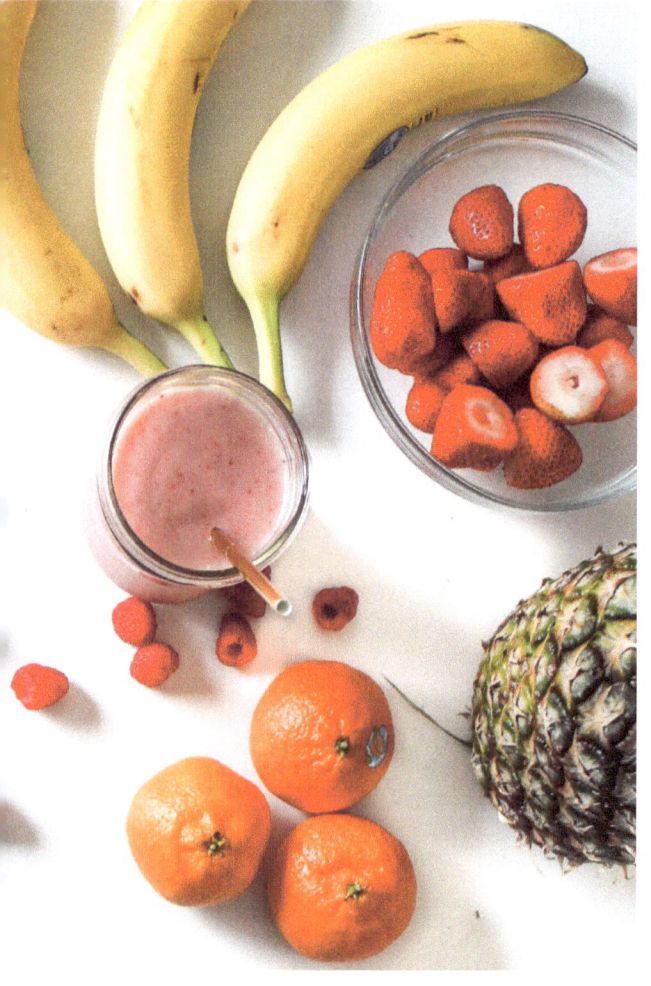

Meal-prepping is a good tool to ensure you are eating food that is good for your total health and weight loss goals.

I like to make my meals look delicious because I believe that we eat with our eyes first. *"Food tastes as good as it looks."* If something looks good before you taste it, you have already signaled to your mind that you like it. Serve your food on a nice plate, and arrange the food on the plate so that it's appealing to the eye. Add color and garnishments.

Be creative. Creativity does not have to be complicated. Mix and match food: eat breakfast food for dinner and dinner for breakfast, Try different food options. Don't assume you don't like something before you try it. Taste buds can be trained like any other senses of the body. Don't underestimate your tastebuds' ability to change. Training your taste buds is a book topic of its own.

Create a Recipe

I provide a list of ingredients below. Maybe something is on the list that you have never tried. Think outside of the box. Maybe something is listed that you tried as a kid and did not like. Remember: Taste buds change. Your mindset can also change. There goes that word *mindset* again.

Your recipe should include sources of protein, fat and carbs. Think about what your body needs. If your medical professional has provided you with a nutritional guide, use the guide to help you create a recipe.

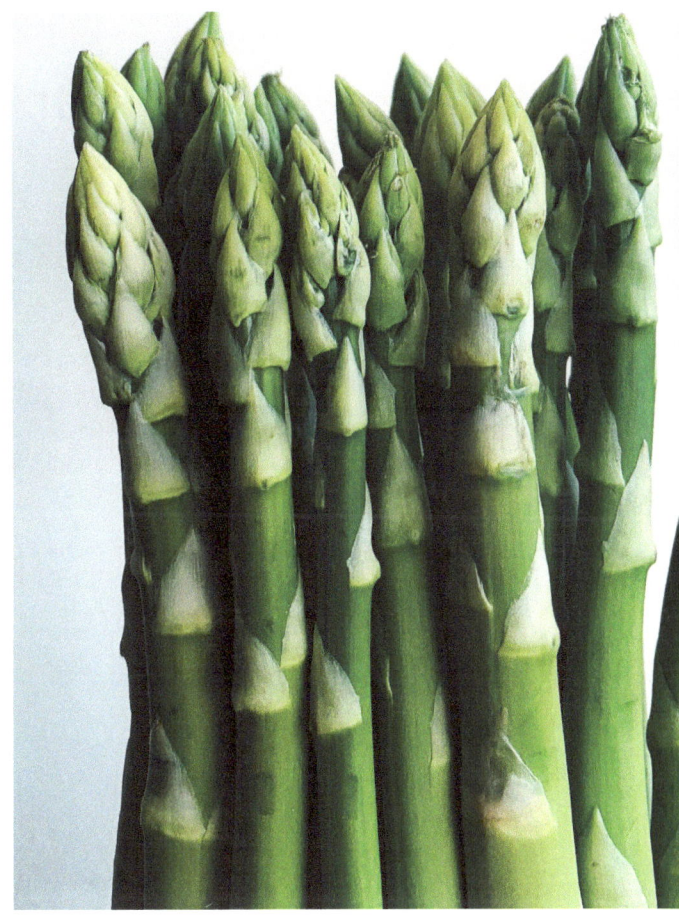

The objective of this exercise is to create a new meal-prep habit that is fun and rewarding. Take this time to learn more about the ingredients on the list below or add ingredients to the list. Here is a little tip: Broccoli can be a protein source as well as a carbs source. Broccoli is a superfood that has fiber, vitamin C, vitamin K, iron and potassium.

FRUITS	GRAINS	VEGGIES	BEANS
Avocado	Oats	Spinach	Lima Beans
Apple	Brown Rice	Mushroom	Lentils
Coconut	Barley	Zucchini	Pinto Beans
Oranges	Farro	Tomato	Chickpeas
Blueberries	Buckwheat	Peppers & Onions	Navy Beans
Strawberries	Teff	Carrots	Black Beans
Banana	Quinoa	Cauliflower/Broccoli	Mung Beans
Pears	Millet	Sweet Potato/Yam	Snow Peas
Mango	Bulgur	Asparagus	Snap Beans

OTHER INGREDIENTS	FATS	ANIMAL PROTEIN
Salt and Pepper	Grapeseed Oil	White Fish
Minced Garlic	Sesame Seed Oil	Eggs
Parsley	Olive Oil	Chicken
Mustard	Nuts	Lean Beef
Hot Sauce	Avocado Oil	Ground Turkey
Crusshed Red Peppers	Coconut Oil	Salmon
Dark Chocolate		
Chives		
Shallots		
Balsamic Vinegar		
Garlic Powder		
Onion Powder		
Curry Powder		

Recipe for: _____

INGREDIENTS

- ✓ _____
- ✓ _____
- ✓ _____
- ✓ _____
- ✓ _____
- ✓ _____
- ✓ _____

PREPARATION

1. _____
2. _____
3. _____
4. _____
5. _____
6. _____
7. _____

> Often time we have everything we need at our *fingertips*.

Core Exercises

A few years ago, I experienced serious back pain. I thought maybe I had pulled something while exercising or cleaning the house. I went to my doctor who referred me to a physical therapist. It was determined that I had a sliding back disc and weak core. My physical therapist prescribed that I strengthen my core muscles as the best method to improve my back pain.

My therapist was correct. As I began to regularly engage in exercises to strengthen my core, my back pain reduced.

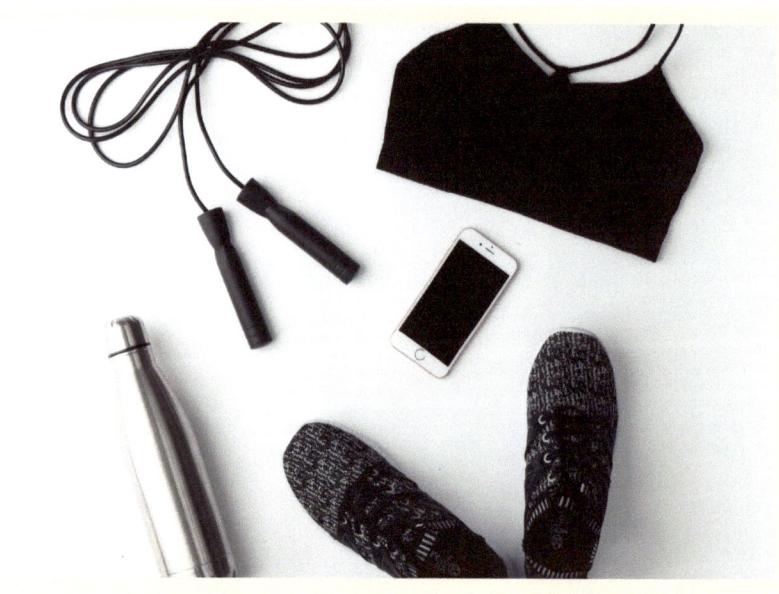

The exercises that I found effective were those that includes, complete core work, work of the transverse abdominal muscles and those that work multiple muscle groups at one time, especially large muscle groups such as legs. Here are three core exercises I do 2 rounds of each exercise, 4 times a week.

Glute Bridges

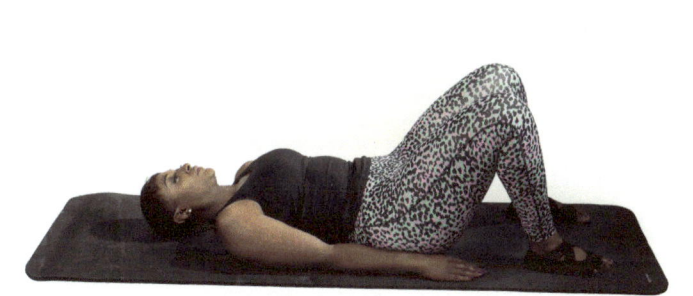

➡ Lay on your back with your knees bent in a 90-degree angle.

➡ Brace your core by drawing your navel toward your spine.

➡ Begin to roll your pelvic area upward while moving your hips toward the ceiling slowly.

➡ Roll your spine upward as well, until your shoulders are about ½ inch off the ground.

➡ **PAUSE FOR 3 SECONDS.**

➡ Then imagine starting the movement from your neck and doing the reverse.

➡ Once you get to your shoulders, start lowering the body down little by little.

➡ Once the movement gets to your hips, repeat from the starting point **20 times.**

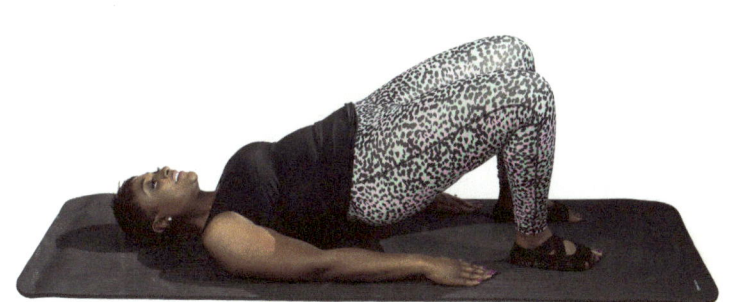

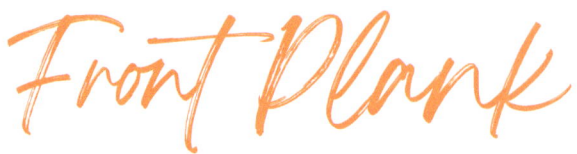

- Get down on the floor onto your elbows and knees.

- Straighten your legs from that position, going onto the balls of your feet.

- Make sure your spine is in a straight line.

- Hold this position for **60 seconds**. If this is too challenging. Lower your knees to the ground and hold a plank position, keeping your spine straight.

- It's important that you do not hold your breath during this exercise.

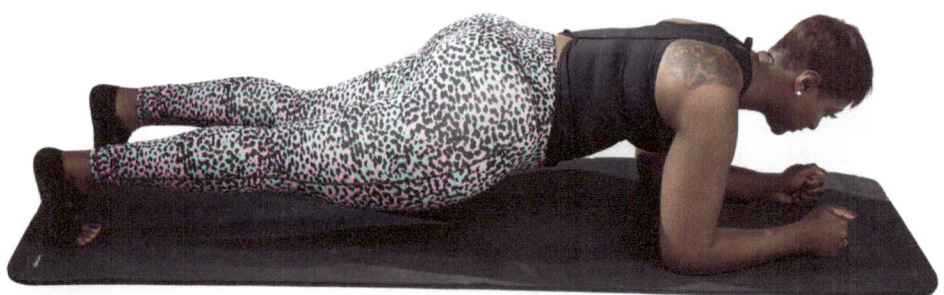

Side-Plank

- Get onto the ground and lay on your side, stacking your hips and feet.

- From this side elbow position, exhale and lift your hips off the ground and knee from the floor.

- Make sure your head and spine are in a straight line.

- Continue to inhale and exhale as you hold the position for **30 seconds for each side.**

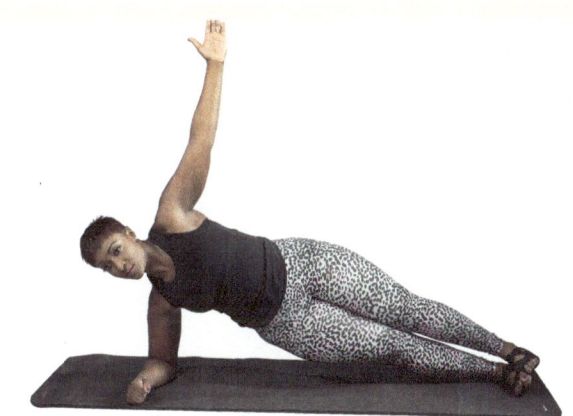

ALTERNATIVE: A less intense option is to

- Get onto the ground and lay onto your side with right knee on top of left knee, right hip on top of left hip.

- Bend the inside knee and lift your hips and knee from the floor.

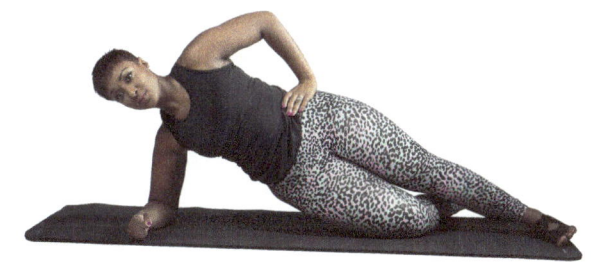

BUFFALO CHICKEN Quesadilla

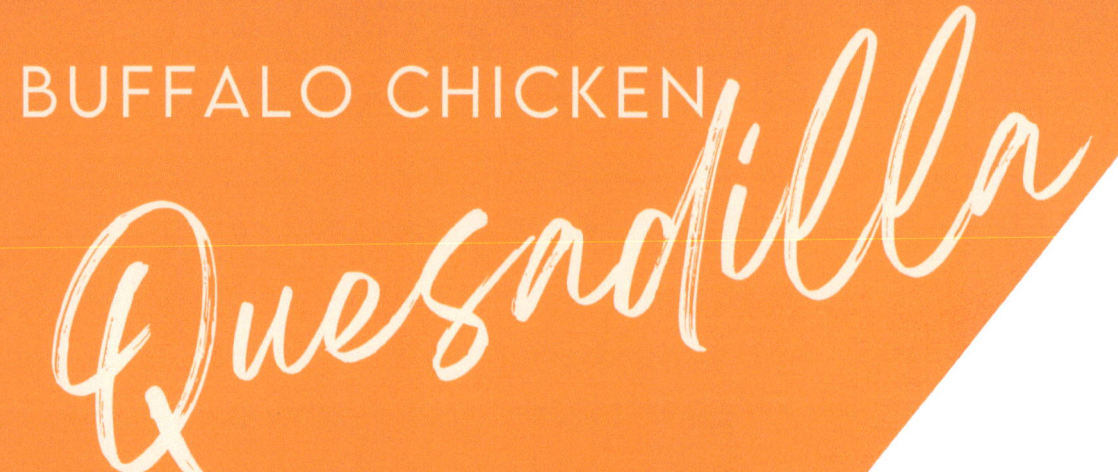

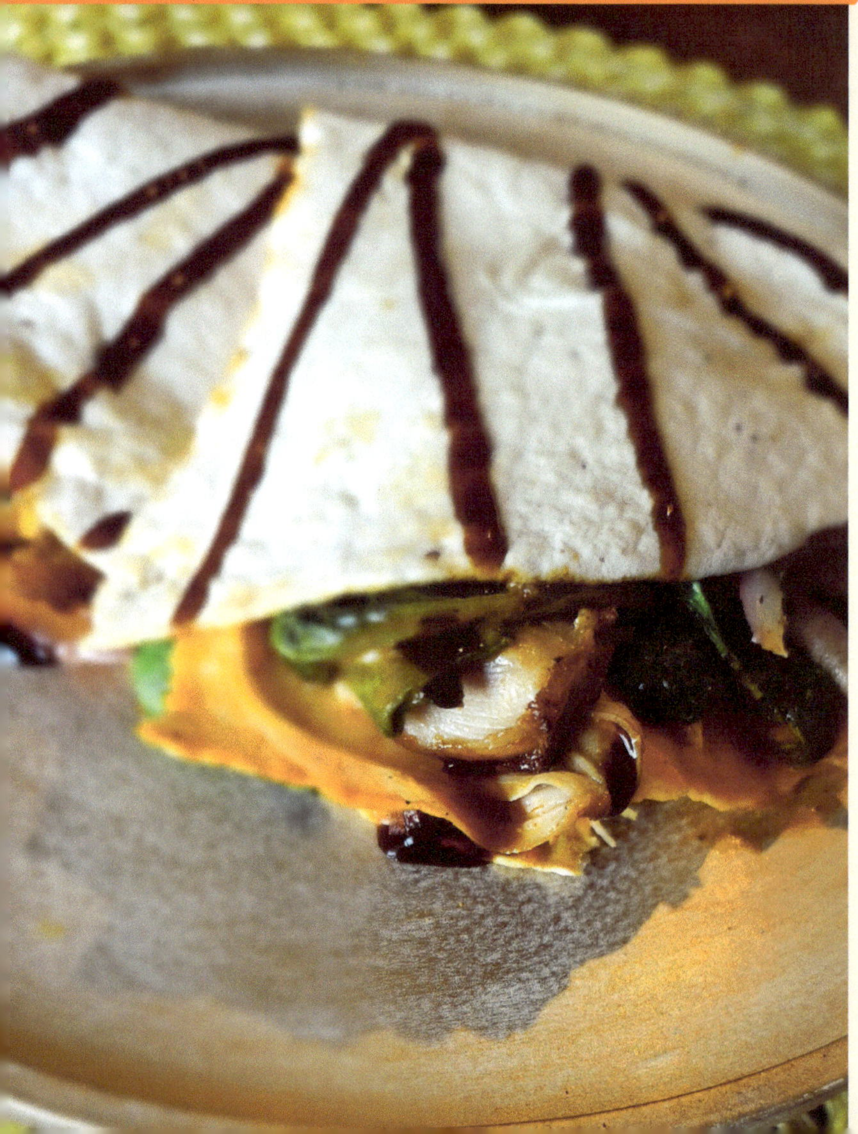

READY IN: 20 MINUTES

SERVING SIZE: 2

INGREDIENTS

- ✓ 8oz Skinless boneless chicken breast, chopped
- ✓ 1 cup Spinach
- ✓ Balsamic glaze
- ✓ Pinch of salt and pepper
- ✓ 1 Red onion
- ✓ 2 Wheat tortillas
- ✓ Olive oil cooking spray
- ✓ Avocado buffalo sauce
- ✓ Mustard
- ✓ 1 Tbsp Garlic powder

PREPARATION

1. Wash all produce
2. Thinly slice red onions and put to the side.
3. Clean chicken and pat dry with a paper towel. Season with salt, pepper, and garlic powder and lightly coat the chicken with mustard.
4. Put the chicken in the air fryer cook for the recommended time for chicken per air fryer instructions. Alternately, you can cook in a large frying pan, flipping every 3 minutes until chicken is thoroughly cooked.
5. Meanwhile, coat a frying pan with olive oil and sauté spinach and red onions to your liking.
6. Once meat and veggies are cooked, put them to the side.

7. Put the stove on medium heat, apply olive oil spray and add 1 wheat tortilla. Spread buffalo sauce on the visible side of the tortilla.

8. Add chicken and veggies on top of half of the tortilla in the pan. Use a spatula to fold the empty half over the meat and veggies. Press the tortilla with the spatula for 45 seconds.

9. Remove tortilla from pan and place on a plate. Add balsamic glaze on the top or serve on the side as a dipping sauce.

Unlock the key to your success by setting your own *expectations for yourself.*

LEAN BEEFY STUFFED *Potato*

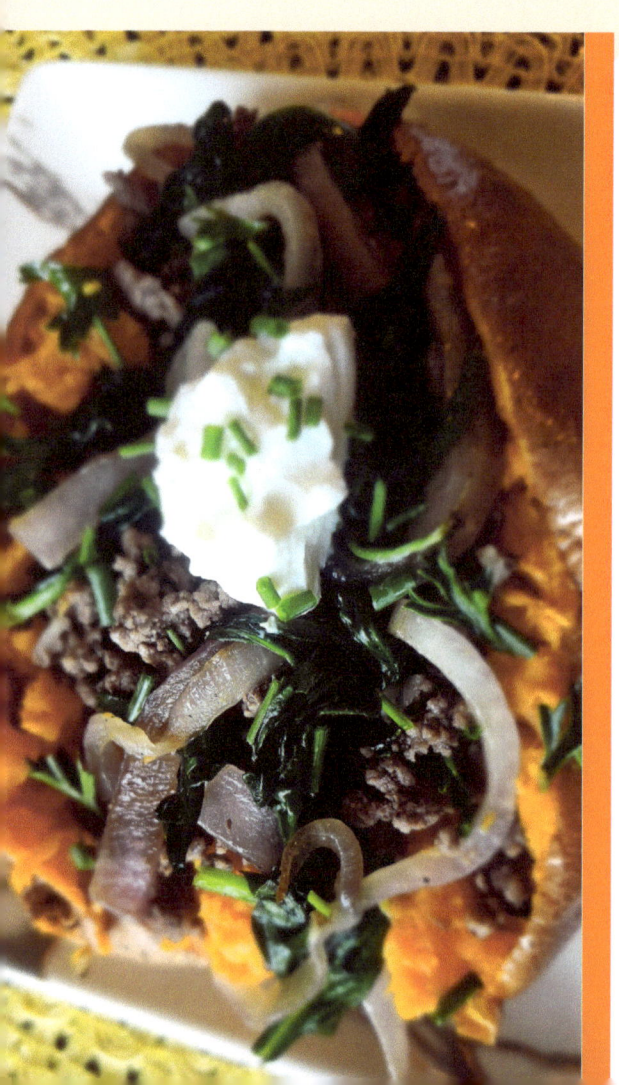

READY IN: 30 MINUTES

SERVING SIZE: 2

INGREDIENTS

- ✓ 3 - 5oz Lean ground beef
- ✓ ½ tsp Sea salt
- ✓ ⅛ tsp Pepper
- ✓ ¼ cup Red onion, chopped
- ✓ 1 tbsp Greek yogurt
- ✓ 1 Medium garlic clove, pressed
- ✓ 1 Potato (russet or sweet potato), washed
- ✓ 1 tsp Fresh parsley, chopped
- ✓ 5oz spinach
- ✓ 1 tsp ground cumin
- ✓ 2 tsp olive oil
- ✓ Fresh chives, chopped

PREPARATION

1. Pierce potato with fork several times, Cook in microwave on high for 7-8 minutes. Set aside to cool for 5 minutes.
2. Meanwhile, in a bowl season lean ground beef (or turkey or chicken) with salt, pepper, ground cumin, parsley, and garlic.
3. Bring a medium skillet to medium heat and add olive oil. Add beef mixture and cook until brown.
4. Add spinach and cook for another 3 minutes. Drain excess liquid. Set aside meat and spinach mixture.

5. Slice the potato in half and scoop potato flesh into a medium bowl, being careful to preserve the skin. Add meat and spinach to the bowl of potato flesh. Then add the potato flesh, meat and spinach back inside the potato skin.

6. Add Greek yogurt and sprinkle fresh chives on top.

TIPS

Beef can be switched out for ground turkey or ground chicken. To add a little southern flavor, swap out spinach for collard greens.

Biological Cravings

I don't know about you, but I am human. I experience both hormonal and physiological cravings. A craving is an urge to obtain something. *Ghrelin is the hormone responsible for stimulating an appetite, promoting fat storage, and increasing food intake.* For example, when my Ghrelin level is high my drive to eat increases and I overeat. *A physiological craving is when I eat because I am stressed, my mood controls my desire to eat.* During my menstrual phrases, I notice an increased desire for food as well. I crave anything that contains sugar. I don't need cake or candy but I do enjoy potato chips. To be honest I just crave food, I enjoy trying different foods. Eating an uncontrolled diet is not good for my metabolism, weight management, or overall health. To balance my hormones is a forever job. I'm not perfect, but I am consistent at making an effective effort. Below are a few things I do to help minimize my cravings and balance my hormones:

1. Drink 80 oz of water a day.
2. Eat every 3-4 hours, balanced meals that include protein, carbs, and fat.
3. 30 minutes of fasting cardio 2-3 times a week. (Exercising on an empty stomach, after 6- 8 hours of sleep.)
4. Strength training for at least 45 minutes 3-4 times per week.
5. Get 6-8 hours of sleep, and take naps when necessary.

NOTE:
Everyone's cravings are NOT the same, and the plan to balance these cravings may vary from person to person. Take the time to understand what your body and mind are asking for. That is the real key to controlling your cravings. **To learn more about your hormone levels, consult with your doctor.**

CRANBERRY OATMEAL *Cookies*

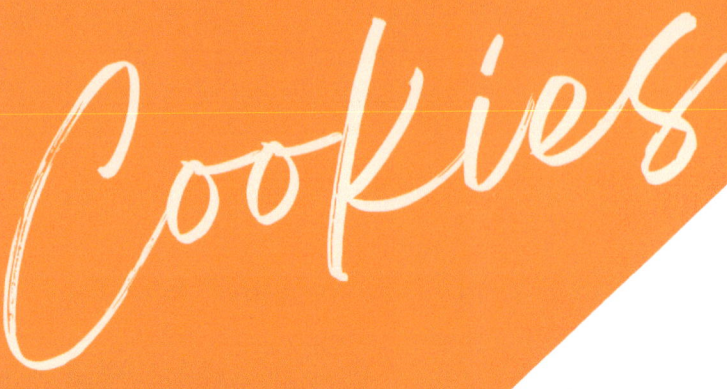

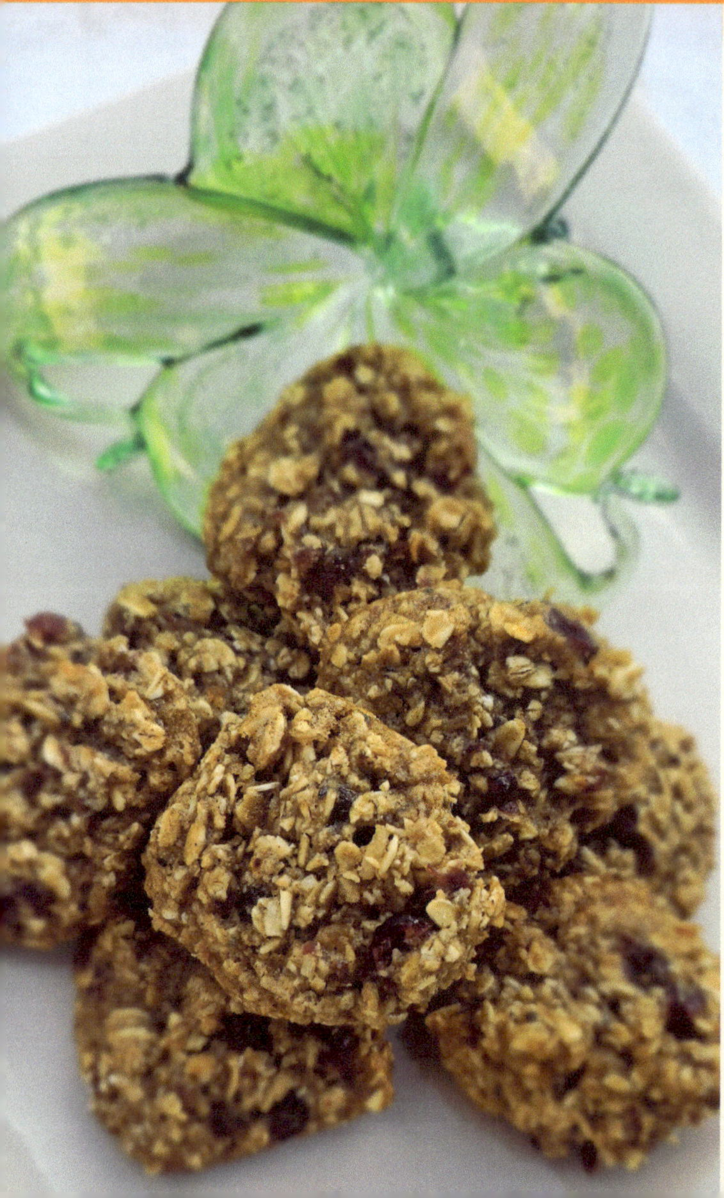

READY IN: 15 MINUTES

SERVING SIZE: 12-14

INGREDIENTS

- ✓ 3 Overripe bananas
- ✓ 2 tbsp agave
- ✓ 1 tsp ground cinnamon
- ✓ 1 tsp ground ginger
- ✓ ¼ tsp sea salt
- ✓ ½ cup dried cranberries
- ✓ 1 ½ cup rolling oaks
- ✓ 1 tsp pure vanilla extract
- ✓ Parchment paper

PREPARATION

1. Preheat the oven to 375°F. Line the pan with parchment paper.
2. In a bowl, mash bananas.
3. Add all other ingredients into a banana bowl and mix into a dough-like consistency.
4. Scoop 1 tbsp of dough onto the pan in rows until no more dough is remaining.
5. Bake for 10 to 12 minutes or until your desired firmness.

TIPS

You can swap cranberries out for raisins or chocolate chips.

Take care of your body and the results will *take care of itself.*

Treadmill Workout

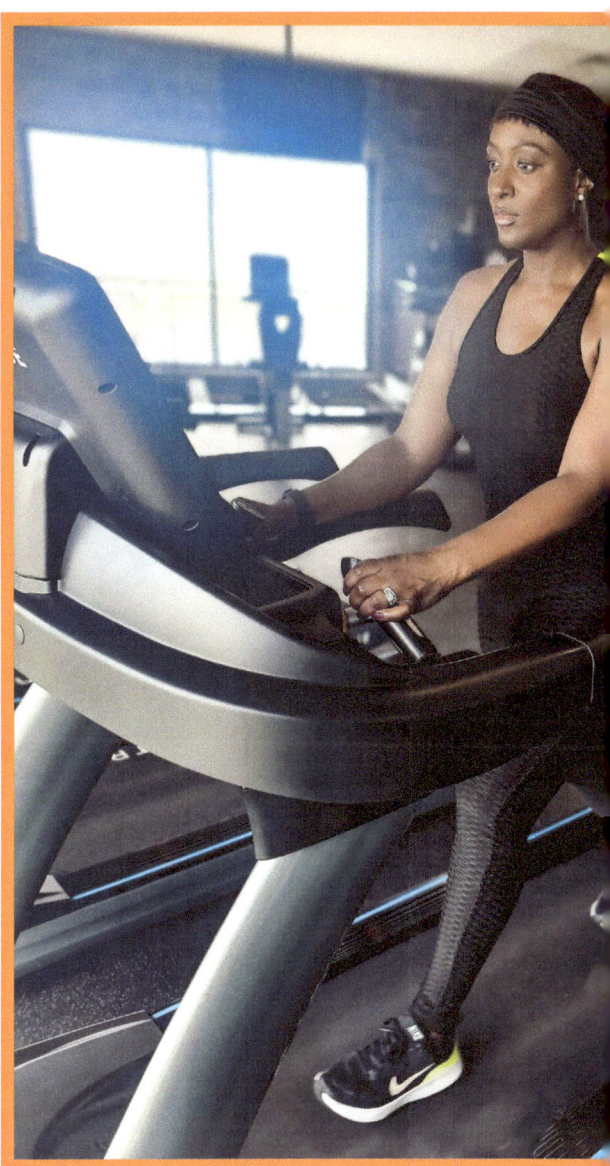

- 5 min moderate pace walk
- 1 min jog
- 20 second walk
- 40 second sprint
- 20 second walk
- 40 second sprint
- 20 second walk
- 40 second sprint
- 20 second walk
- 40 second sprint
- 20 second walk
- 40 second sprint
- 10 min incline speed walk
- 5 min jog
- 5 min cool down walk

Tip: If you can't jog or sprint, walk at the fastest speed that you can, I've noticed a great improvement in my speed and endurance by doing this treadmill workout 3-4 times a week.

SMOTHERED BONELESS CHICKEN &... *Veggies*

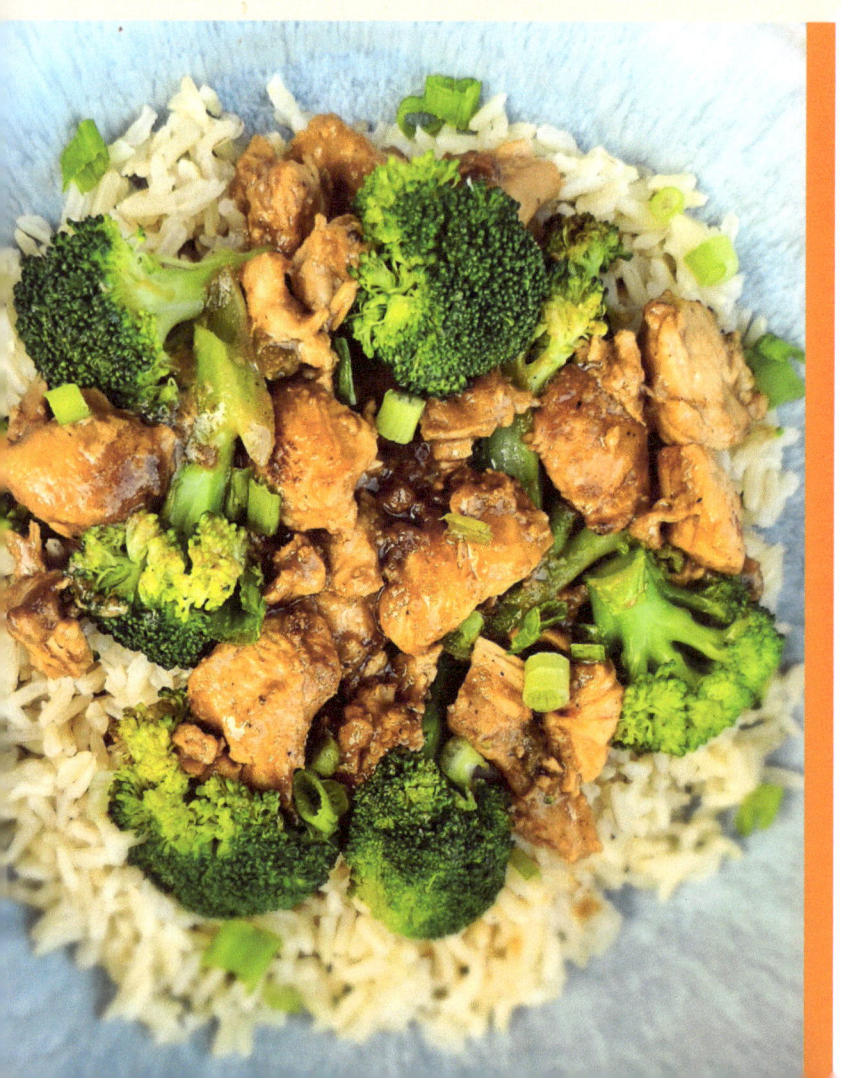

READY IN: 20-30 MINUTES

SERVING SIZE: 2-3

INGREDIENTS

- ✓ 10 oz Boneless chicken breast pieces
- ✓ ½ cup Brown rice
- ✓ ½ lb Fresh broccoli
- ✓ 2 Scallions
- ✓ 1 tbsp Balsamic vinegar
- ✓ 2 tbsp of Soy sauce
- ✓ 1 tbsp Sesame oil
- ✓ 1 tbsp of Organic agave
- ✓ 2 tbps of Chickpea flour
- ✓ 1 tbsp of Water
- ✓ Garlic powder
- ✓ 1 tbsp Sherry vinegar

PREPARATION

1. Clean chicken.
2. Use a paper towel to pat the chicken dry. Then season chicken with garlic powder, salt, and pepper.
3. In a bowl mix sherry vinegar, balsamic vinegar, and chickpea flour. Stir until chickpea flour is dissolved. Add seasoned chicken to bowl of mix and stir until chicken is coated.
4. Cook brown rice by following rice bag instructions and add a pinch of sea salt.
5. Wash all produce.

6. Cut off about ½ off bottom of broccoli stem, then cut broccoli into medium to small florets and put to the side.
7. Thinly slice scallions, separating green top and white bottom.
8. In a bowl combine balsamic vinegar, soy sauce, sesame oil, agave and tablespoon of water making a sauce.
9. Heat a pan to medium–high heat and add a drizzle of olive oil. Add broccoli florets and season with salt and pepper. Add white bottom of Scallions and ¼ of water. Loosely cover the pan with aluminum foil and cook. When finished, transfer to a bowl.
10. In the same pan broccoli was cooked, add chicken and cook on both sides until lightly brown. Now add sauce and cook for about 2 minutes. Once done, turn off the heat.
11. Finally, serve over brown rice, chicken, and broccoli.

Minus the inconsistency

this journey is not that bad.

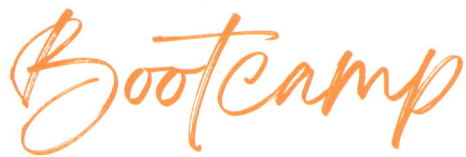

Bootcamp

Let's talk about my favorite type of exercise. I enjoy participating as a member of bootcamps. I enjoy boot camp because it allows me to maintain endurance and build muscle. I love how boot camp motivates me.

The things I look for in a good boot camp are knowledgeable trainers, team-oriented energy, great music, and exercises that challenge my body and mind. I've had the pleasure of being a member of some awesome boot camps in Orlando, Florida.

IS BOOTCAMP AN EXERCISE PROGRAM YOU WILL LIKE?

1. Do you like exercise that is in a group setting?
2. Do you want to build muscle?
3. Do you like to do different exercise moves?
4. Are you looking for an exercise program that will challenge you?

If you answered yes, to at least three of these questions, you may like a bootcamp style exercise program.

HOW TO FIND A GOOD BOOTCAMP:

1. Do the bootcamp demonstrate alternative moves for different exercises?
2. Do the bootcamp offer morning and evening sessions?
3. Encourage teamwork?
4. Are the trainers knowledgeable?
5. Offer 30 min-45 min sessions and 50-60 min sessions?
6. Is nutrition guidance available?
7. Does the boot camp incorporate warm-up movements as a part of the session and cool down stretching after session?

Always consult with a medical professional before beginning any exercise program.

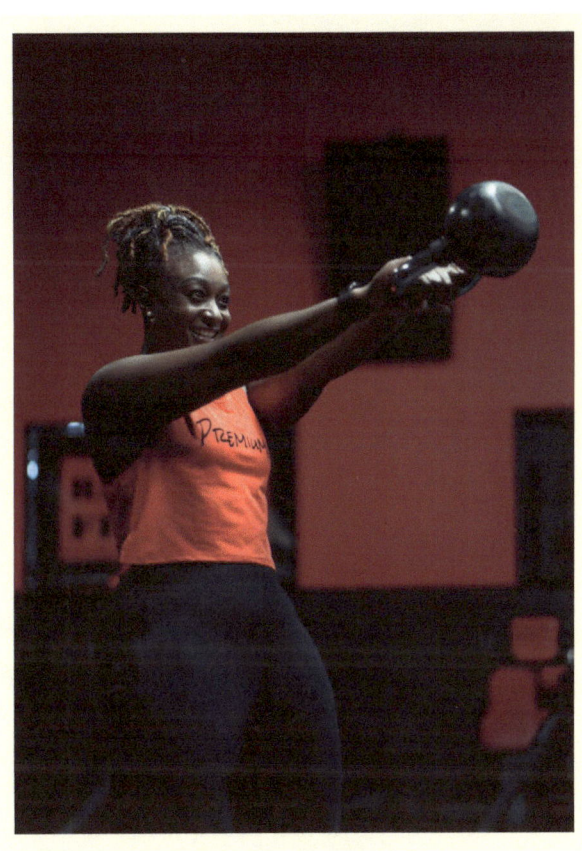

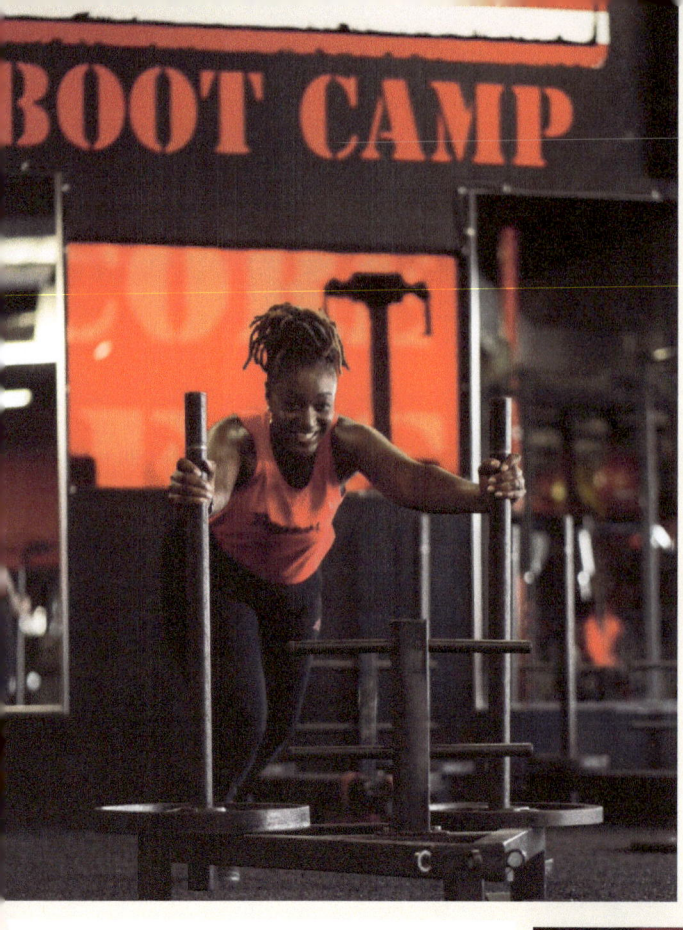
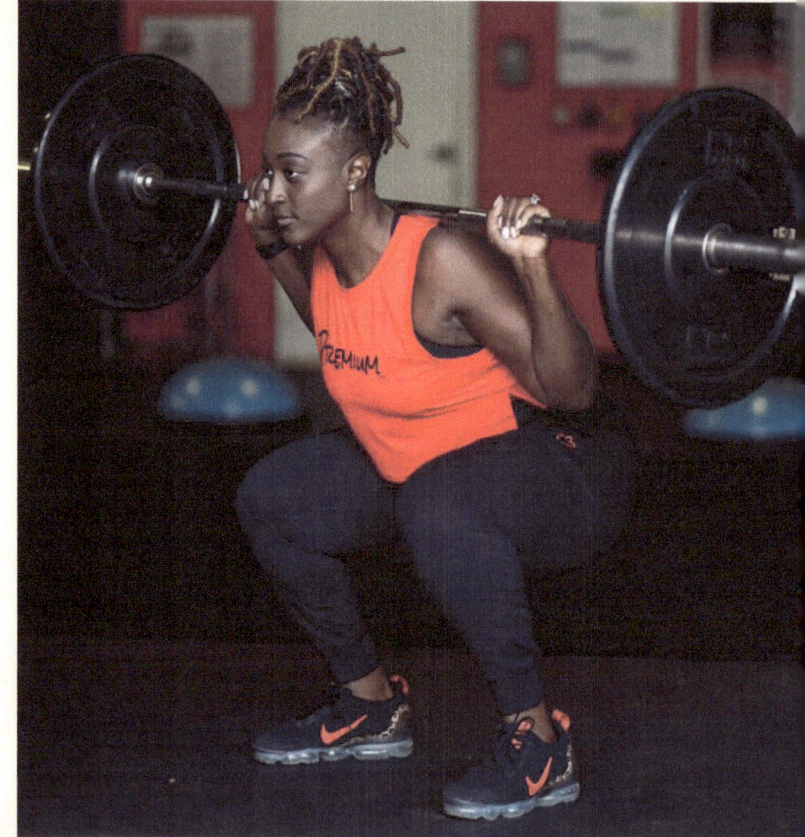

WHEN TIME IS LIMITED BUT I NEED TO MAKE SURE I HAVE AN ACTIVE DAY HERE ARE A FEW THINGS I LIKE TO DO:

- ➡ Walk for 10-15 minutes during my lunch or other breaks.
- ➡ Park the furthest from the door at work.
- ➡ Use the restroom that is the furthest, including on a different floor level.
- ➡ Complete 10 squats every time I go to the restroom. (I always go the restroom furthest away.)
- ➡ Use stairs instead of elevators.

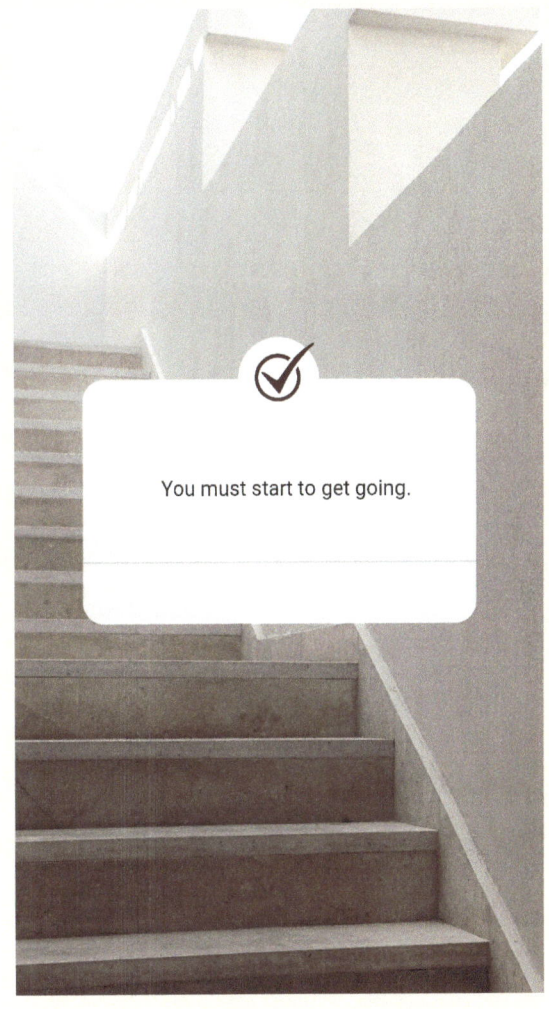

You must start to get going.

PUMPKIN SEEDS & ALMONDS
Roasted

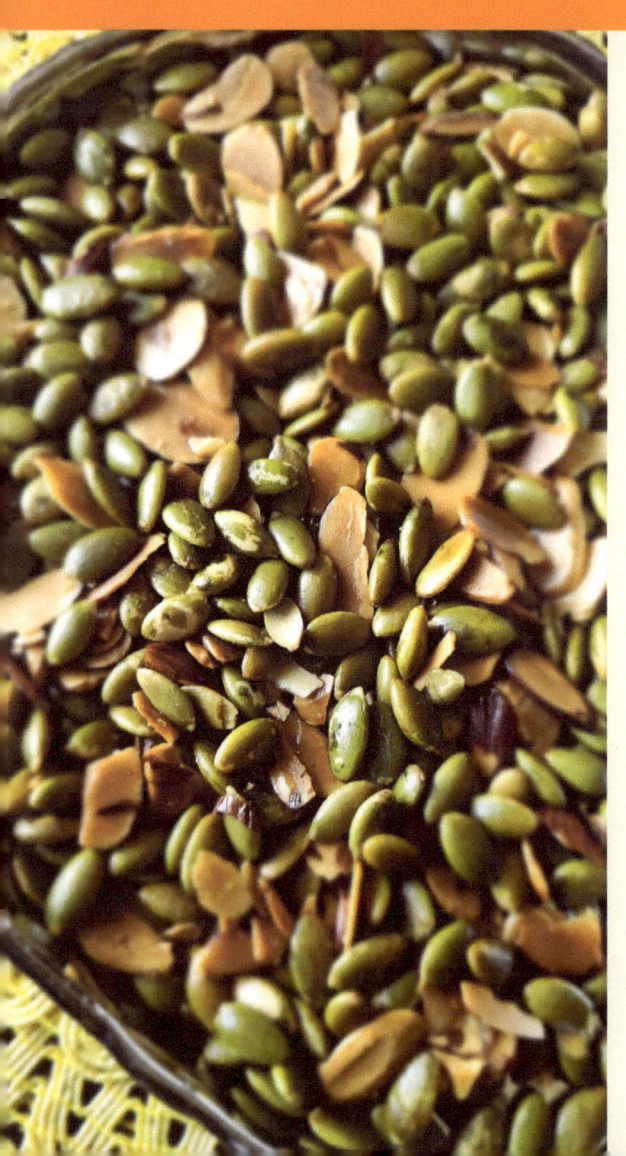

READY IN: 25 MINUTES

SERVING SIZE: 1-2

INGREDIENTS

- ✓ ¼ cup of Pumpkin seeds
- ✓ ¼ cup of half Slice almonds
- ✓ 1 tbsp Olive oil
- ✓ 1 tsp Sea salt

PREPARATION

1. Preheat the oven to 300°F.
2. Toss seeds and nuts with olive oil and salt.
3. Arrange seeds and nuts mixture in a single layer on a baking sheet.
4. Roast/bake for 15-20 mins. Check the seeds and nuts mixture every 10 mins and stir them around.

TIPS

Store roasted seeds and nuts mixture in an airtight container at room temperature. I like to eat pumpkin seeds and sliced almonds as a snack. I literally eat one nut/seed at a time, to trick my mind into thinking that I am eating a lot. I also like to drink ½ cup of oak milk with this snack.

Choices

As I've gotten older, managing my weight has gotten more challenging. This could be due to age, hormones, life, or a combination. As the mother of a teenage athlete, I am always busy. I'm also a very active sister, daughter, wife, friend, and manager. Therefore, I had to change my focus to eating food and exercising for total health.

I prioritize eating essential food and exercising as normal activities in my life rather than for seasons or special occasions. Eating greens and fruit is not a challenge for me because I understand the benefits of eating these foods. Exercising does not feel like a chore to me because it makes me feel good inside and out.

This perspective shift of no longer seeing eating well and exercising regularly as chores was a game changer for me. Making better food choices and exercising can also result in weight loss, but there are other benefits. I look forward to exercising. It is often a joyful part of my day. I compare how I feel when I don't consume essential food to how I feel when I do and oh, what a difference! I feel less bloated and sluggish. I think clearer and my skin glows.

> Let's be clear, I don't make the best food choices all the time. I enjoy eating food. I also don't categorize any food as *bad* food. However, it is a fact that some foods have more benefits than others and too many foods that have negative effects on the body have negatively affected mine. Therefore, I choose to make better food choices and give my body what will have positive impacts more often than not.

Life is like a recipe:

The measurement is based on a serving.

SWEET AVOCADO *Salsa*

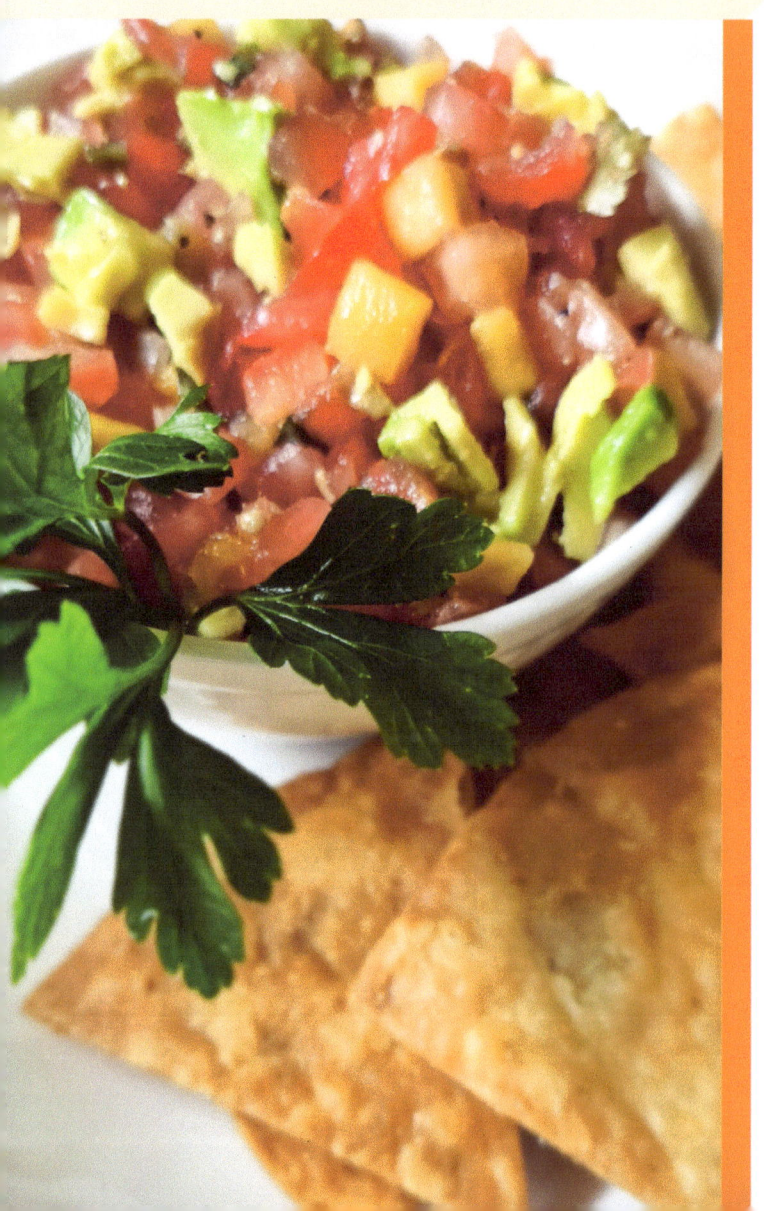

READY IN: 5-7 MINUTES

SERVING SIZE: 2

INGREDIENTS

- ✓ 1 Large avocado, diced
- ✓ 1 Large mango or 1 ½ cup of pineapple
- ✓ 1/3 of Cherry tomatoes
- ✓ 2 tbsp Red onion, finely chopped
- ✓ 2 tbsp Fresh cilantro, chopped
- ✓ ½ tsp of Sea salt
- ✓ 2 tbsp of Green onions, finely chopped
- ✓ ½ tsp of Apple cider vinegar
- ✓ 1 tsp Garlic, diced
- ✓ 3 tbsp of Fresh Cilantro leaves
- ✓ 3 tbsp of Fresh lime juice

PREPARATION

1. Cut mango/pineapple into small cubes and put in a large bowl.
2. Chop cilantro leaves and place in a bowl with mango.
3. Put red and green onions in a bowl with mango.
4. Slice tomatoes into ¼ small pieces and place in a bowl with mango/pineapple.
5. Add garlic powder, vinegar, lime juice, and salt and pepper to taste.
6. Combine all ingredients. Let chill in the refrigerator for 15 minutes or you can eat at room temperature.
7. Serve.

TIPS

The Sweet Avocado Salsa is a great mid-day and late-night snack!

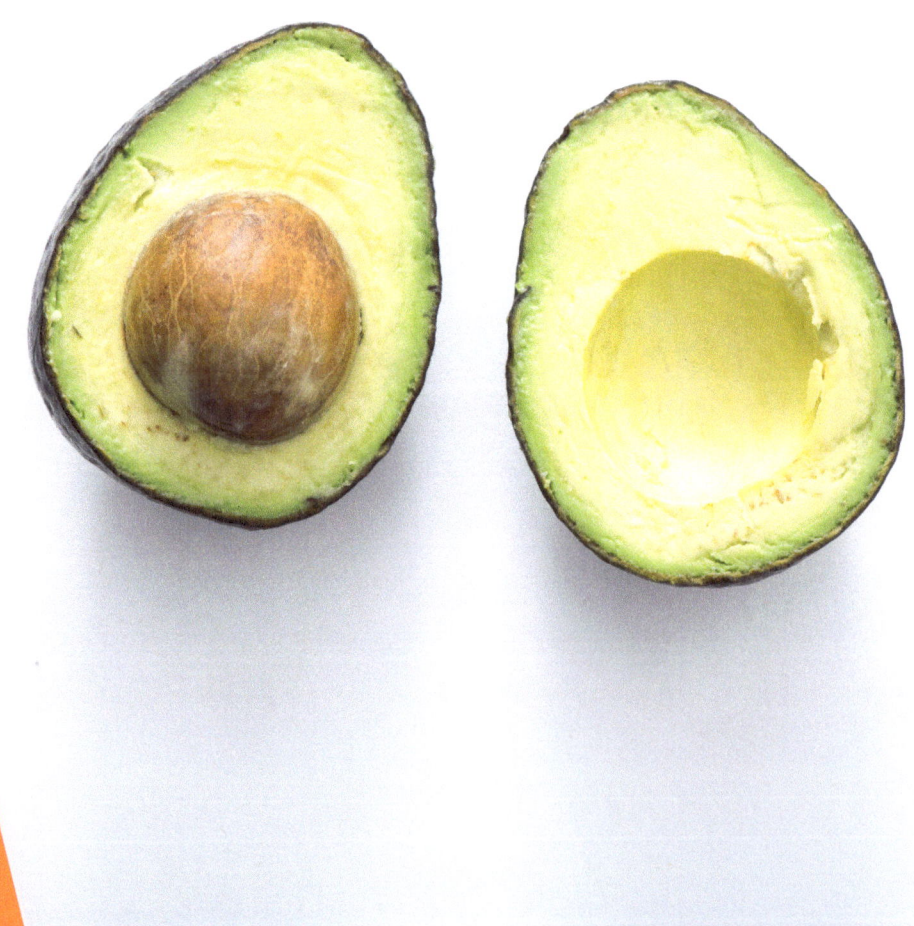

Tips I Use for Vacation

ENJOY: If not what is the point?

MOVE: I try to exercise, dance or go for a walk at least 30 minutes a day.

DON'T OVEREAT: I do not starve myself and I eat before I get hungry. I eat smaller meals. This allows my body to carefully process the food, reducing sickness, miserableness, and sluggishness.

BE INTENTIONAL: Eat a fruit and/or vegetables daily.

BE MINDFUL: Be mindful of my sugar intake and consume it wisely.

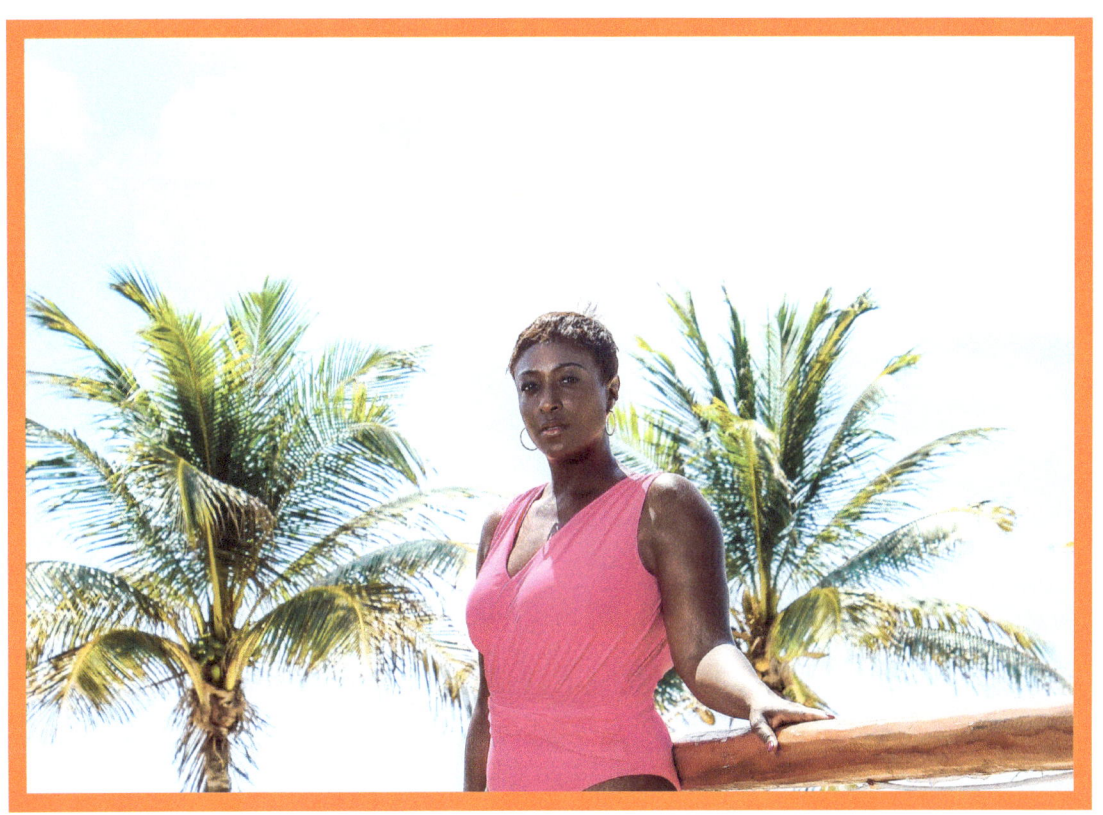

CUCUMBER & CITRUS INFUSED *Water*

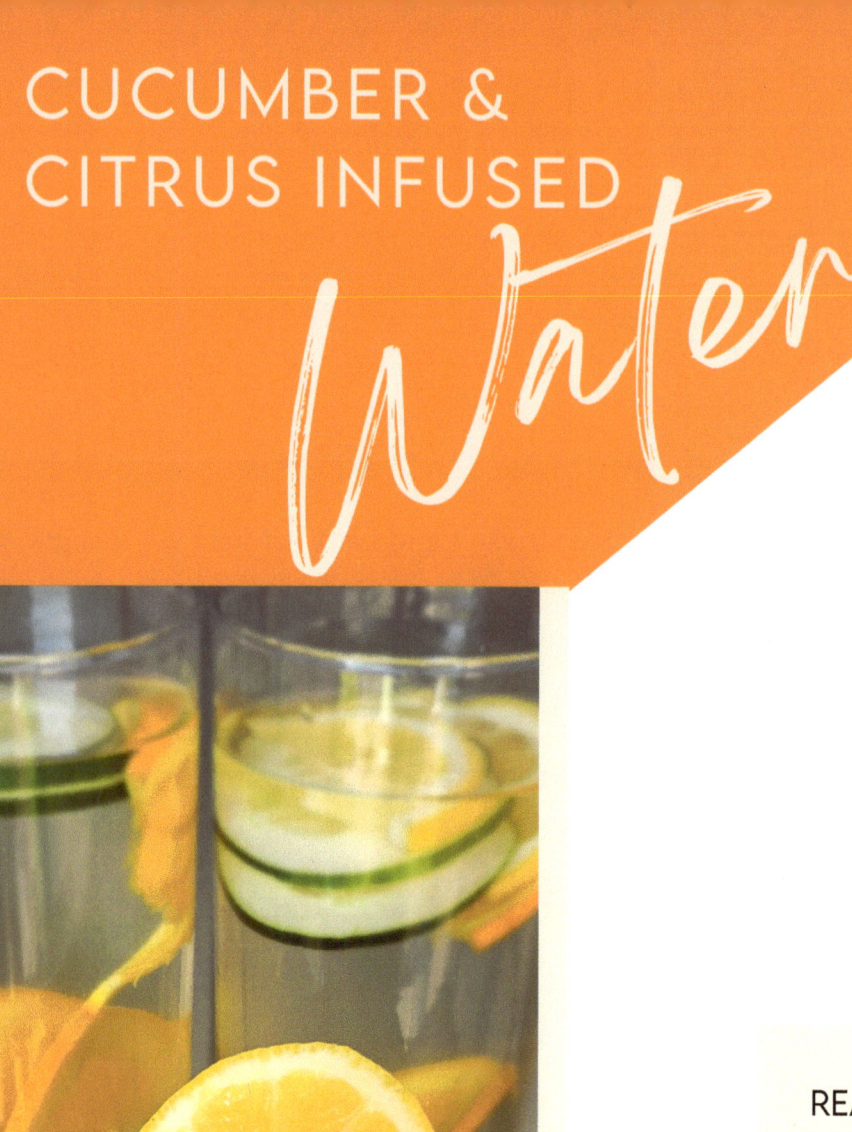

READY IN: 1 HOUR

SERVING SIZE: VARIES

INGREDIENTS

- ¼ of Lemon
- ½ Cucumber
- ¼ Orange
- 1 gallon Alkaline water
- *Optional:* mint

PREPARATION

1. Slice fruit and put it into the gallon of water.
2. Chill in the refrigerator for one hour.

TIPS

If you are in a rush, infuse cold water and place in the refrigerator for 10 minutes. The longer it is infused the stronger the taste will be. Removal of rind from lemon and orange will reduce bitter taste.

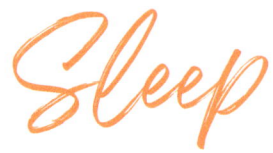

Sleep

When you sleep, you rest. Rest is a time for your body and mind to recharge. Good sleep is essential for my health, and I notice that when I get quality rest, I have more energy in the day. Additionally I can focus better throughout day. I strive for 6-8 hours of sleep nightly, and one 10–15-minute power nap a couple of times a week.

TIPS TO AID A GOOD NIGHT SLEEP

1. 5-20 min of stretching before bed.

2. I drink water before bed. My skin looks so refreshed in the morning. *Note: Because I hydrate all day long, drinking water before bed does not make me go to the bathroom more frequently than if I do not drink water before bed. The amount varies depending on the person. Consult with your doctor and find the amount that works best for you.*

3. No TV or phone use for 30 minutes before getting into bed. I use this time to do box breathing. Box Breathing is a breathing technique also known as 4-square breathing. Here is the short version of the steps.

    I. Inhale slowly through the mouth, count to 4.

    II. Hold your breath for a count of 4.

    III. Exhale slowly for a count of 4.

    IV. Repeat.

BOX BREATHING TECHNIQUE

✓ Sit up with a comfortable straight back. Close your eyes, inhale-exhale normally for 10 seconds to clear your mental pathway.

✓ Then start box breathing after an **exhale-inhale** slowly through your nose while counting to four.

✓ Next hold your breath for another count of four, avoid clamping down on your teeth.

✓ Now slowly breathe out through your mouth for a count of four.

✓ After exhaling, hold your breath for a count of four.

✓ Repeat this breathing pattern as you desire.

Psalm 4

"In peace, I will lie down and sleep, for you alone, Lord, make me dwell in safety."

Fall asleep to the comforting promise of Psalm 4, as you name and lay your worries down at God's feet —

one by one

From the Author

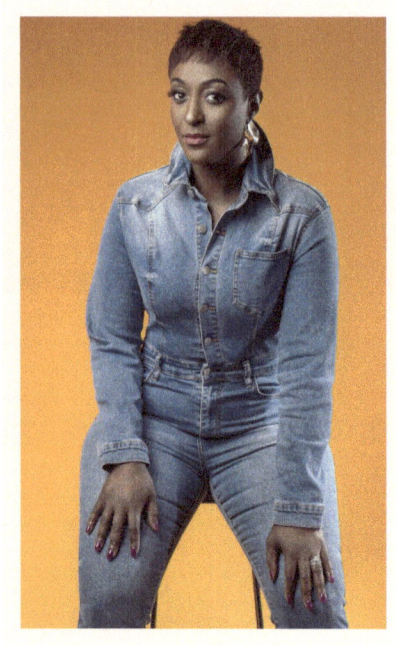

I hope you enjoyed this book. I found so much joy in sharing within this book ways I've learned to love myself. Happiness starts with self-love. To truly love yourself includes taking care of yourself to the best of your ability. I understand the trials of balancing life. I have downfalls like everyone else. I know so well how easy it is to fall back into unhealthy habits. But I also know the peace of feeling good inside and out. So, I challenge anyone who has read this book to hold me, you, a friend, a family member, a coworker, or a stranger accountable and encourage them to demonstrate self-love. Let's do this together accountability works.

GET SOCIAL WITH ME
Instagram | Threads | Facebook | TikTok **@hypetobefit**

VISIT
www.hypetobefit.com for free tips, recipes, workouts, and more.

TAKE THE CHALLENGE
Send a random letter, email, or text to someone sharing with them what you like about them and share something you learned from reading this book.

Together we can strive to live a life of love and purpose-driven as God intended.

www.ingramcontent.com/pod-product-compliance
Lightning Source LLC
Chambersburg PA
CBHW040724060526
44119CB00083B/319